MACROBIOTICS AND BEYOND

MACROBIOTICS AND BEYOND

Marcea and Daniel Weber

AVERY PUBLISHING GROUP INC.
Garden City Park, New York

This book is dedicated to my son Elijah
who gave a new meaning to the word 'Macrobiotics'.

First published in Australasia in 1988 by
Nature & Health Books,
This edition co-published in Great Britain by
Prism Press, 2 South Street, Bridport,
Dorset DT6 3NQ, England

Copyright © 1988 Marcea and Daniel Weber

All rights reserved, no part of this publication
may be reproduced, stored in a retrieval system,
transmitted in any form or by any means, electronic,
mechanical, photocopying, recording or otherwise,
without the prior permission in writing of the publisher.

ISBN 0-89529-445-1

Design: Craig Peterson

CONTENTS

Acknowledgements	7
Introduction	9
Food and Cookery Terms; Australian and American Equivalents	14
Macrobiotics — Then and Now	15
Recipes:	
Winter	21
Spring	35
Summer	48
Late summer	62
Autumn	73
Cold desserts	84
Fresh fruit desserts	87
Tarts, puffs and other sweet delights	90
Cakes	97
Cookies, biscuits and bars	102
Breakfast recipes	109
Beverages	121
Stocks and standard marinade	123
A word on rice — storing, preparing and cooking	129
A Total Approach to Well-Being	133
Yin and Yang Diet	141
Kitchen-Wise	145
Chinese System of Diagnosis, Treatment and Foods	153
Actions of Foods in the Seasonal Recipes	163
Foods and Their Associated Organs, Energies and Flavours	168
Suitability of the Recipes for Various Diets	173
Alternative Ingredients for Restricted Diets	187
Alternative Sweeteners	189
Equivalency Chart Metric Conversion Charts	191
Glossary	195
Where to Shop	203
Bibliography	205

Tao produced the One,
The One produced the two.
The two produced the three.
And the three produced the ten thousand things.
The ten thousand things carry the Yin and embrace the Yang
and through the blending of the Ki they achieve harmony.

Tao Te Ching

ACKNOWLEDGEMENTS

We would like to thank our friends, who supported us throughout the writing of the book; our students who shared their experiences, questions and desire for 'more'; our teachers Michio and Aveline Kushi, Cornelia and Herman Aihara, and Masahiro Oki, who were always willing to listen to our questions and then sent us out into the world to discover our own truth.

Many thanks to our dear friend Janet Donald, for your support, fine knowledge of cooking, editing and typing; to our dear friend Catriona Macmillan, for your positiveness, support and inspiration; to another dear friend, Sandra Lawry, who entered our lives just at the right moment like a gift from heaven and who collated all the Chinese information of foods and their action, nature, meridians and organs, and who gave form to the book.

Thanks also to our dearest friends Jan and Dan Rowan for your support and faith, and for your willingness to share our son with us when we needed more time and space than we thought was possible; to another dear friend, Suzie Wright, for your initial support and trust; and to many other friends and spirits who nurtured us along the way.

Marcea and Daniel Weber

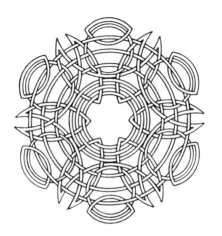

INTRODUCTION

I recall a question that one of my students once asked me, after I had finished teaching a Yoga class. It had to do with my views about the relationship between diet, health and fitness. I brewed it over in my mind for a few seconds before I responded, then muttered something about 'macrobiotics' being the perfect panacea and watched the person's face suddenly shift from inquisitiveness to confusion. I guess I was so anxious that everyone I met be converted on the spot (or at least that they would acknowledge and support me) that I didn't even take into consideration whom I was speaking to. I tried very hard to explain the philosophy and make her 'get it' that moment, using words like 'Yin and Yang' without realising that she hadn't a clue as to what they meant (let alone how to apply them). So instead of being interested she just became increasingly removed, disinterested and withdrawn.

I learned a lot from that incident, and gradually stopped trying to impress people that I met. I began to study the philosophy of macrobiotics and apply it in my daily life.

It's now considered a fact medically that food has a profound effect on our physical and emotional well-being. And while this recognition extends historically to the Greeks, for example, in our modern culture it is a very recent innovation. In 1969, when we were in Boston studying Macrobiotic philosophy, the Food and Drug Administration raided a health food shop and confiscated books that claimed food could cure disease and that it had some definite effect on health. The FDA claimed that everybody knew that food had no effect on health or disease. So, in reflection, we can see that in just a few short years, things have shifted dramatically.

Only since the end of the nineteenth century have people looked into the quality of food and into the combining of food, especially where it concerns vegetarians. Before that time people were mostly concerned with having enough to eat, and with having a reasonable variety of foods to eat. They were also interested in the cleanliness of the food: was it uncontaminated, was it unspoiled? Now, of course, it is acknowledged that food affects our well-being.

In the Orient, this understanding has been relevant since the Han dynasty in China, between the second century B.C. and the first century A.D. when a number of works were written on dietetics (the medicinal use of food). From the period between the Han period and the Tong period which lasted 800 years, forty major works on diet and nutrition have survived. In the *Su-Wen*, a collection of essays on medicine from the first century A.D. we find the following quotation: 'It's an

MACROBIOTICS & BEYOND

example of how dietetic treatment, as opposed to drug therapy was assessed. The Chinese understood the more potent the drug, the smaller the range of illnesses could be treated, whereas dietetic therapy could be applied almost against any affliction . . . Medicinally potent drugs can eliminate six out of ten illnesses. Drugs without marked medicinal effectiveness (such as food), can eliminate nine out of ten illnesses. Grains, meats, fruits, and vegetables are suitable for dietetic nourishment against all illnesses. But even with these certain limits should not be exceeded. Otherwise the proper (influences) of the (patient) might be harmed.'[1]

So the history of dietetics in the Orient is just as long as ours, but more importantly has been included into the training programme of physicians, whether they be practitioners of Chinese herbalism, Acupuncture or Western medicine. A Chinese physician was always concerned about the combination of foods for each individual person, taking into consideration the seasons, weather and personal items. A medical specialist in dietetics was known as a *shih-i*, and people with this role are described in the following way: 'Their task is to care for the balance of the six food stuffs, six drinks, six dishes, hundred provisions, hundred soups, and eight precious dainties of the king. When they prepare rice dishes the (warmth of) springtime should be taken as an example. When soups are prepared, the (heat of) summer should serve as an example. When they prepare sauces, the (coolness of) fall should be taken as an example. When they prepare drinks, the (coldness of) winter should be taken as an example.'[2]

Also, the Oriental system relied upon flavours, recognising that certain flavours enhance certain functions of the 'depots' or organs, so not only was care taken in the preparation, but in the balance of flavours, emphasising particular flavours for certain conditions. The thermal property of a food was also taken into consideration. Certain foods were considered to be warming or cooling, so these were all included. This is a very different proposal from Western scientific nutrition, where mainly molecular components of food are considered. The Orientals, especially the Chinese, were more concerned with the 'energetic' component of food. Food that is grown naturally, without the use of artificial chemicals or pesticides, and tended with care, will provide all the nutrients necessary. But the quality of the food was and still is important, especially if one wants to maintain a healthy and balanced state of being.

Medical practitioner and Author Sun Ssu-mo (581-682 AD) is quoted as saying 'For the human body to remain in a healthy and balanced state nothing else is required but to care about its nourishment. By no means should drugs be consumed recklessly. The strength of drugs is one-sided, and there are occasions where they are

1. Lung Po-chien. *Hsien-ts 'un pen-ts' ao shu-lu*, Peking, 1957, p.48.

2. Lung Po-chien. *Hsien-ts 'un pen-ts' ao shu-lu*, Peking, 1957 p.48.

I N T R O D U C T I O N

of help. But they lead to an imbalance of the influences in man's 'depots' and consequently, an affliction will easily be acquired from outside (sources). Living beings have always-depended on food to maintain their life. But, at the same time, they are unaware of the fact that even food has positive and negative aspects. (Food) is in daily use with all the people, but one knows little about it.'

The author goes on to say that practitioners of medicine must first of all recognise the origin of an illness; 'They must know which violations (have caused the suffering). Then they must treat it with dietary means. If dietary therapy does not cure the illness, only then can they employ drugs. The nature of drugs is violent, just like that of imperial soldiers. Because the soldiers are so wild, how could anybody deploy them recklessly? If they are deployed inappropriately, harm and destruction will result everywhere. Similarly, excessive calamities are the consequence of drugs thrown against illnesses (carelessly).'[3]

As I mentioned earlier, the Chinese divided food into energetic properties. The two most common aspects were flavour and thermal influence. In their traditional concept of *Yin* and *Yang* (balance and harmony) certain flavours were considered more *Yin* while others were considered more *Yang*. Certain temperatures were also more *Yin* or more *Yang*. Overall, however, flavour was the more *Yin* influence, and temperature the *Yang* influence. So the combination of certain flavours with certain temperatures gave rise to the basics of energetic nutrition.

The basic flavours were sour, bitter and salty, which were considered the most *Yin*. Spicy, sweet and neutral were considered to be flavours having a *Yang* property within the *Yin*. The temperatures warm, hot and balanced were considered *Yang*, while cold and cool were *Yin*. So the primary quality of food from *Yin* to *Yang* would be: cold/sour, cold/bitter, cold/salty. A bit more *Yang* would be balanced/sour, balanced/bitter, balanced/salty. Moving to the thermal influences, food could range from being mostly *Yang* — warm/spicy, warm/sweet, hot/spicy, hot/sweet — through to *Yin* and *Yang*. This was still *Yang* but with a *Yin* property: cold/spicy, cold/sweet, cold/neutral, cool/spicy, cool/sweet, cool/neutral. These flavours were also affected by the seasons, particular 'depots' or organs of the body, and the influence of thought and well-being.

So when we look at Chinese dietetics in relationship to Western nutrition, in terms of its content, vitamins, minerals, proteins, fats, complex carbohydrates it may even seem a bit antiquated and even perhaps a little superstitious. When we are talking about these energies, we are talking about metaphors that we experience directly. It requires no training, for example, to experience ourselves being hot or clammy. On the other hand, in Western nutrition, the assessment is a technical, objective one. You have to have a label, a name like 'penumonia', in order to present

---

3. P.U. Unschuld, *Medicine in China*, University of California Press, 1986.

MACROBIOTICS & BEYOND

an appropriate drug. If a person has a fever, heavy cough or thick mucus, in Western Medicine we have to take a sample of the sputum in order to know whether this is bacterial, viral or an environmental problem to do with dust or asbestos. We wouldn't know until we tested it thoroughly, and when it was tested the appropriate medicine could be prescribed.

However, when it comes to eating, it seems silly to make a daily or weekly pilgrimage to an expert, to find out what it is that we should be eating. Certainly, if we seek out expert advice and receive an opinion, then this is only a guide and that's all.

We use it and when we feel the need to change and adapt our diet once again according to our own needs we should remain flexible enough to do so.

In the basic experiential medicine of the Orient, we notice, we see, we listen, we look, and by observing in these ways we can tell exactly what it is that we have to do. We strive always to produce harmony and balance. For hot disease states, we take more cool or cold foods, (never totally one or the other, since we should always use a little of the opposite to make balance); for damp we take more drying foods, for energies that rise, we take foods that 'descend'. When we understand the principles of internal/external, hot/cold, dry/damp, deficient/excess, and *Yin* and *Yang*, and also the various qualities of the flavours, and we then incorporate them into our way of life, it becomes very easy to match specific foods to specific disease states (not withstanding the need sometimes for professional medicine). In this way we take more responsibility for ourselves and for our family's well-being.

Macrobiotics, derived from Chinese dietetics, is one of the most essential diets which supports us in finding out what it is we need, and when. Once we master some of the very simple ground rules and understand and appreciate some of the very simple movements of energy such as *Yin/Yang*, the flavours, the thermal properties and the 'energetics' of food, it then becomes more simple for us to use food on a daily basis to maintain health and well-being, prevent disease states and in some circumstances even cure diseases.

The influence of all this is made possible by a sense of inner wisdom, knowing on the deepest level, and seeing through the direct experience of that. This is the highest level of Macrobiotic medicine and healing. Through understanding food and its properties we have a great capacity to alter a condition that may be impairing our well-being. So, in a way, Macrobiotic medicine — or the simple medicine of experience — is actually the 'people's' medicine. It is something that takes place in families, it is something that takes place in communities amongst friends and associates. It is something that we have for ourselves, notwithstanding the importance of conceptual medicine and the training that has to be done. We respect doctors, whether they be engaged in herbalism or surgery. We respect their expertise, however, by returning some responsibility to ourselves. To become well

12

I N T R O D U C T I O N

in ourselves through our own means is an important first step to healing the community as a whole.

It is our profound wish that you, the reader, use this book as a guide and support system in preventive health care and learn about your individual needs, thus taking more responsibility for your own wellness. The bottom line is that you should really learn to enjoy what you do and what you eat. This is not intended to be a cookery book; it is merely meant to supply an explanation about the nature and energies of foods — what they are made of and how they can be transformed through unique preparation and cooking to support you.

Macrobiotics and Beyond is meant to be a companion to other cookery and books on health and is to be used in conjunction with them. Use the charts at the back of the book with other recipes that you may fancy and create meals that suit your own individual needs. Our goal is to bring together the cuisine of East and West and an ancient way of looking at harmony for our own well-being that works in this day and age. By recognising the differences and similarities of each individual culture and ourselves we can learn many things, and only by our own experiences will we truly gain a deeper appreciation and respect for our own extraordinariness.

Marcea and Daniel Weber

FOOD AND COOKERY TERMS:

Australian and American equivalents

Australian	American
grill	broil (except when cooking outdoors)
biscuit	cookie
filter	strain
prawn	shrimp
shallot	scallions
capsicum	red pepper

MACROBIOTICS — THEN AND NOW

The foundations of macrobiotics were laid in the seventeenth century. Ekken Kaibara, born in 1630, eight years before Japan began to shut itself off from the rest of the world, greatly influenced philosophies concerned with health and well-being. He was attracted to classical Chinese philosophy and became a leading figure in the Neo-Confucian School. To the original teaching of Confucianism, the 'new' Confucianists added Taoist ideas about how the universe began and how it should function. The central philosophy of the Taoists was the Tao Te Ching ('The Way and Its Power'), in which the universal absolute 'Tao' or 'Oneness' was seen as having expression in two complementary yet opposite energies, Yin and Yang (later to be further identified as Male and Female). From the Tao all things were created and manifested according to the Order of the Universe, and all things were and are constantly changing and moving. Kaibara wrote several books which embraced this view of life. One of these books, Japanese Secrets of Good Health, suggests that sickness, like health, is something that we create: it comes only when one has wilfully abused oneself, never occurring without reason.

Taoists view the human body as being similar to the Earth, with skeletons corresponding to mountains, orifices to valleys, and blood vessels to rivers. Thus it seems natural that everything which occurs inside us is part of the same process occurring in Nature and its surroundings. So just as other facets of Nature have to adjust to climatic and seasonal changes, we too should adjust our inner forces — such as our emotional, glandular and spiritual states — with the external forces of Nature. As the conditions and seasons change (hot, cold, damp, dry, humid, wet), the balance of energies between our diet, work, relationships, exercise, activity, sex, thoughts, meditation and sleep should reflect and be dependent upon Nature.

Kaibara makes some suggestions regarding the choice, preparation and manner of eating food; these include:

— Eat rice as a daily staple food.
— Eat fresh vegetables when they are in season.
— Eat simple light meals of foods that are clean, freshly prepared, peaceful in quality and balanced in terms of the five tastes, sweet, sour, salty, bitter and pungent.
— Avoid hard and fatty meat. Some lean poultry and game may be eaten sparingly.
— Fish should be eaten whole if possible, and cooked with ginger and soy sauce in order to neutralise poisons.
— Above all, do not overeat. Eat only 80-90 per cent of capacity, until just before one feels full.

MACROBIOTICS & BEYOND

— Before eating, remember with gratitude the farmers and others who have produced the food, the parents and benefactors who have supplied it, and those who have cooked and served it. Remember too, those who are without food, and one's unworthiness before such blessings.

— Never eat while angry or worried.

— Do not eat before going to bed.

— After eating take a short walk to stimulate circulation. Massage the stomach and the abdomen lightly to encourage circulation.

Kaibara's other thoughts include:

— Physical exercise and the cleansing of mind and heart thus gained are essential to health.

— Do not expect too much of others.

— Through the working of Heaven and Earth we are an integral part of Nature.

Ishizuka Sagen, born in 1850, was the next main figure in the history of macrobiotics. Just as Western medicine was being introduced into Japan, he moved to Tokyo and began to work and study in a hospital there. He eventually became an allopathic doctor. Unable to cure a chronic kidney condition which resulted in a serious skin inflammation, he began to look at traditional Oriental medicine, particularly the ideas presented in the Yellow Emperor's classic text. He conducted a vast number of experiments on himself by fasting on certain foods, a month at a time, and noting the effects. Ishizuka is responsible for developing the theory that a proper balance in the body between the salts of sodium and potassium can determine the body's ability to absorb and utilise other nutrients. His basic conclusion was that human health and sickness depend on diet above all. He believed that good food improperly prepared can lead to illness, and that nutritionally unbalanced foods (such as meat and eggplant) can be made more balanced by adding certain foods. It was also his belief that the choice of an appropriate diet should also include consideration of personality traits, physical characteristics, psychological patterns and spiritual conditions.

Yukikazu Sakurazawa, later known as George Ohsawa, discovered the works of Ishizuka and was responsible for bringing this philosophy (Shoku-Yo, as it was called by Ishizuka) to Europe and America under the name of Macrobiotics. Ohsawa also believed that food plays a critical role in human lives, determining a person's degree of health or sickness, happiness or sadness, physical appearance, behaviour and moral and spiritual sensitivity. He attempted to fuse Western scientific approach with traditional Japanese and Chinese medicine by combining the concept of acid and alkaline with the Oriental philosophies of Yin and Yang.

According to Ohsawa, health is a state of balance between the forces of Yin and

MACROBIOTICS

Yang. As everything in life is relative, flexible and changing, it is up to us to judge what is appropriate at any given time. For example, in the winter when cold (Yin) forces dominate the environment the body requires extra warming (Yang) energy, which may be gained through hot food and vigorous exercise. In order to keep the body and mind in a state of balance, it is best to maintain yourself with preventive care such as proper diet and exercise, and to pay attention to the changes in the weather, season, geography and emotional condition.

Herman Aihara and Michio Kushi are two men who have furthered Ohsawa's teachings in the Western world. With the support of Ohsawa, Michio Kushi came to the United States with the aim of studying world peace and spreading macrobiotic philosophy and the teachings of Ohsawa. Herman Aihara also discovered George Ohsawa's teachings, and later emigrated to the United States where he worked with Michio Kushi to establish macrobiotics. The two men expanded the body of macrobiotic thought to include ideas on world government and peace, meditation and diagnosis of health problems. Acceptance of the diet was very slow, but today many people in the United States and other countries throughout the world practise macrobiotics in their daily life.

NEW AGE MACROBIOTICS

Macrobiotics has taken the brunt of most anti-vegetarian criticism, even though it isn't considered to be vegetarian in its approach or philosophy. Many nutritionists condemned the so called 'macrobiotic diet' of the late 'sixties and 'seventies as a dangerous dietary fad, and the American Medical Association coined it a 'major health problem'. These viewpoints were based on data that the diet contained too many carbohydrates, fruits and vegetables, and not enough eggs, fish, poultry, meat and dairy products, as well as including very little if any sugar, margarine or butter. Now, the Australian Nutrition Foundation has put out a pamphlet titled 'Eating For Health And Pleasure', in which it states that the more cereals, wholemeal and mixed grain bread, vegetables and fruits the better, and advises people to have less cheese, milk, yoghurt, lean meat, legumes, poultry, fish, nuts and eggs, and an even smaller amount of margarine, butter, oil and sugar. Basically, it's about having more fibre and less fat in our diets.

Many people have the wrong idea about healthy eating. They think that it means giving up all enjoyable foods. It is worth mentioning here the words of a friend of mine who described his own personal experience with macrobiotic diet and philosophy as such: 'It's not what I thought it would be like at all. Sometimes brown rice doesn't even enter into the picture; sometimes macrobiotics has virtually nothing to do with diet or brown rice. Macrobiotics is a way of life, a philosophy, that

17

some people discover by changing their diet, or visa versa. It emphasises balance and harmony, a positive state of mental, emotional and physical well-being'.

Taking an even broader view, here is a dedication written by Michio Kushi.

"When we eat, let us reflect that we have come from food which has come from Nature by the order of the infinite Universe, and let us be grateful for all that we have been given.

When we meet people, let us see them as brothers and sisters and remember that we have all come from the infinite Universe through our parents and ancestors, and let us pray as One with all of humanity for universal love and peace on earth.

When we see the sun and moon, the sky and stars, mountains and rivers, seas and forests, fields and valleys, birds and animals, and all the wonders of Nature, let us remember that we have come with them all from the infinite Universe. Let us be thankful for our environment on earth, and live in harmony with all that surrounds us.

When we see farms and villages, towns and cities, arts and cultures, societies and civilisations, and all the works of man, let us recall that our creativity has come from the infinite Universe and has passed from generation to generation and spread over the entire earth. Let us be grateful for our birth on this planet with intelligence and wisdom, and let us vow with all to realise endlessly our eternal dream of One Peaceful World through health, freedom, love and justice.

Having come from being within, and going towards infinity, may our endless dream be eternally realised upon this earth, may our unconditional dedication perpetually serve for the creation of love and peace, and may our heartfelt thankfulness be devoted universally to every object, person and being."

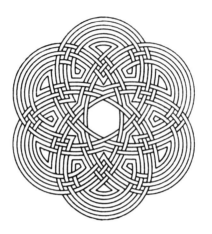

RECIPES

WINTER

Most of my friends and family do not seem to embrace winter with the same gusto or romance as they do spring and summer, or even autumn for that matter. However, winter is, in fact my favourite time as the need to raise one's spirit gets more demanding as the solstice approaches.

Emotionally many people feel much more erratic during winter as it is often time for journeying inward and being more sensitive. Almost everything rests or sleeps during the winter, withdrawing energy from deep within, or from the earth in preparation for the forthcoming season of rebirth and regeneration. Winter is a time for spending more time at home with one's family and friends — resting, reflecting, restoring and being more aware and sensitive to the elements. Around 20-21 June, the date of winter solstice, is considered the first day of winter. It is also the day of the longest night; after that day the hours of light increase and energy begins to gradually build momentum towards spring.

According to the Chinese system, winter is related to the element Water which is contained in the air, and is a part of all living matter. An essential medium of the body, water is vital for eliminating waste and fighting off infections, circulation of the blood, lymphatic flow, urine, saliva, tears and perspiration. Water is nourishing, refreshing and energy-producing. Both the human body and the Earth's surface consist of 70-80 per cent water. As a matter of interest, blood plasma and sea water are somewhat similar. In addition, the two organs associated with winter and the element Water are the kidneys and the bladder, which deal with the body's water supply, elimination and circulation. Because these organs are associated with winter, the Chinese believe that they are actually nourished by the cold climate, but if the cold or dampness is too extreme it is no longer beneficial. It's also important to keep your body dry and warm, especially on the very cold or damp days, because cold conditions can create stiffness in the body.

The taste associated with the element Water is salty. Although salty foods have been somewhat controversial over the past few years, it is a fact that most water is quite salty, and even the water in our body contains many mineral salts. One indication of a water imbalance is a craving for salt. However, eating too much salt creates a desire to drink too much water — which can injure the kidneys and bladder.

There are emotional imbalances occurring all the time in our lives, but the one that is associated with Water imbalance is fear. It could manifest in any one of a number of ways. General anxiety about life, phobias, negativity or paranoia, trembling, or even the blocking of love can reflect some kind of fear.

The kidneys take care of the life force in the bones and marrow, storing it for a time when it is needed. People with bone problems often have a Water imbalance. This would include the skull, spine and teeth as well as the bone marrow, where cells are produced and used for growth and renewal in our bodies. Another delicate balance can be seen in the energy flow during sexual relations. Sometimes problems like infertility or impotence have been known to be related to Water imbalances.

The time of day also affects the flow of energy and different organs in turn. Bladder time is from 3-5 p.m. and kidney time is from 5-7 p.m. If you repeatedly have a difficult time during these hours of the day it may be an indication of Water imbalance. If you have a balanced Water element, then the ability to rest and relax, giving nourishment to yourself and others, is very evident.

Cooked whole grains make a good staple during the winter as they are complex carbohydrates which provide the body with adequate fuel; they also support the intestines by providing fibre which aids assimilation and elimination. Combining beans and grains together in one meal will boost the protein in your diet.

If you are inclined to eat more animal food in the winter, fish is a good choice as winter is related to the Water element. Ocean fish, low in fats with high amounts of protein, minerals and vitamins, are a very good secondary food source. Sea vegetables like kelp, arame and hiziki, are high in minerals such as calcium, iron, potassium, iodine and phosphorus. They provide good nourishment for the hair, skin and nails, and aid the endocrine system.

Because much energy is stored in the roots of plants during the winter season, boiling up some herbal roots can be especially beneficial. They are good blood cleansers as well as tonics. The more common roots traditionally used during the winter months include comfrey, which helps support the lungs and mucous linings (however, comfrey is now listed as a poison by some health authorities in Australia) and ginger root, which helps circulation, stimulates the stomach and aids digestion.

Nourish yourself during these cold, dark months; keep yourself warm, and balance your outward energy-expanding activities with quiet, energy-accumulating, reflective practices like yoga, breathing exercises, meditation and relaxation. Many of Nature's creatures hide during the winter season, gathering energy to emerge once again in the spring. Pamper yourself and explore your inner feelings so that your own rebirth is powerful, vital and complete.

W   I   N   T   E   R

Winter Menus

1 Spinach Garlic Soup
  Parsnip Pie

2 Baked Fish Rolls with Tofu Filling
  Broccoli with Black Bean Sauce

3 Broccoli Cauliflower Mousseline
  Spiced Chickpeas with *Mochi* Topping
  Snow Pea *Arame* Salad

4 Split Pea Soup
  Carrots in Orange Juice
  Buckwheat with Fennel, Onions and Mushrooms

5 Layered Vegetable Casseroles
  Endive, Radish and Mandarin Salad

NOTE: The menus in this book serve 4-6 people.
T = tablespoon
t = teaspoon

Winter Menu 1: Spinach Garlic Soup
                     Parsnip Pie

SPINACH GARLIC SOUP

¼ CUP OIL
4 SLICED GARLIC CLOVES
1 CUP SLICED ONIONS
1 CUP CHOPPED CELERY
½ CUP GRATED PUMPKIN
4 CUPS STOCK OR WATER
3 CUPS PACKED FRESH SPINACH LEAVES
MISO (¾-1 t PER PERSON) OR SEA SALT TO TASTE
TOASTED SESAME SEEDS FOR GARNISH

Forward planning: *Prepare stock. Toast sesame seeds for garnishing.*

1 Heat dry wok or skillet, add oil and sauté the sliced garlic until it is golden. Add the sliced onions and sauté until they turn transparent. Stir in the celery and pumpkin and sauté until they are almost soft.

2 Transfer the ingredients to a larger pot if necessary and add the stock. Bring to the boil, lower the heat, partially cover and simmer the soup for about 5 minutes. Purée the soup until it is smooth.

3 Blanch the spinach leaves by plunging them in and out of boiling water. Drain and chop them finely. Reserve 2 T for Menu 2. Add them to the soup and simmer for another 3 minutes. (If using sea salt season here and simmer).

4 Dissolve the required amount of miso in a small amount of stock; spoon some miso into each bowl and ladle the soup over it.

6 Garnish with toasted sesame seeds.

PARSNIP PIE

Pastry

2 CUPS WHOLEMEAL PASTRY FLOUR
½ CUP GROUND NUTS
1 t DILL SEEDS, CRUSHED
½ t SEA SALT
$^1/_3$ CUP OIL
½-$^2/_3$ CUP BOILING WATER

Filling

4 CUPS THICKLY SLICED PARSNIPS
2 EGG YOLKS
GRATED RIND OF 1½ LEMONS
JUICE OF 1½ LEMONS
2 T MAPLE SYRUP
1 t CINNAMON OR ½ t GROUND GINGER
2 EGG WHITES

Baking equipment: *20 cm oiled pie dish or flan ring*

Forward planning: *Parsnips may be cooked and puréed in advance, and heated through for further preparation. Preheat oven to 180°C.*

Pastry

1 Combine flour, nuts, seeds and sea salt in a bowl. Beat boiling water vigorously into oil until creamy. Add to dry ingredients all at once. Knead the mixture until the

| W | I | N | T | E | R |

dough forms a ball, adding a little more flour or water if necessary. Wrap the dough well so that it does not dry out and leave it in the refrigerator for 15 minutes.
2 Roll the pastry very thinly on a sheet of greaseproof paper and invert over the oiled dish or ring, positioning the pastry to line the dish or ring evenly. Finish edging. Partially bake the crust on the middle rack of a 180°C oven for 10 minutes.

Filling
3 Pressure cook or boil the parsnips until they are tender. Drain and purée them until smooth.
4 Beat the egg yolks with rind of 1 lemon, lemon juice, maple syrup and spice. Stir into the parsnips.
5 Fill the crust with the parsnip mixture and smooth over the top. Bake the pie at 180°C for 15-20 minutes.
6 Remove and lower the heat to 120°C. Beat the egg whites with the remaining lemon rind and a pinch of sea salt until they are stiff. Spread the mixture over the pie. Bake the pie at 120°C for 15-20 minutes or until the top is nicely browned.

Winter Menu 2: Baked Fish Rolls with Tofu Filling
Broccoli with Black Bean Sauce

BAKED FISH ROLLS WITH TOFU FILLING

6 FISH FILLETS OF SIMILAR SIZE
SEA SALT
3 T OIL
3½ CUPS THINLY SLICED LEEKS
1 CUP TURNIPS, CUT IN JULIENNE STRIPS
¼-½ CUP DRY WHITE WINE OR RICE WINE
250 g MARINATED PRESSED TOFU
2 T BLANCHED, WELL-DRAINED, FINELY CHOPPED SPINACH
2 T DICED ONIONS, SHALLOTS OR GINGER ROOT
2 T SOAKED, STEMMED, DICED *SHIITAKE* MUSHROOMS
2 T GROUND SEEDS OR NUTS
¾ t SEA SALT
FRESH CORIANDER LEAVES FOR GARNISH

Tofu Marinade *see recipe next page*
Baking equipment: *A baking dish that will fit the fish rolls in one layer*

MACROBIOTICS & BEYOND

Forward planning: *Marinate the tofu for several hours, then drain and press under a plate for ½ hour or so before using it. Reserve the marinade. Oil the baking dish. Preheat the oven to 190°C.*

1 *Wash the fish fillets and rub them all over with sea salt. Leave for 5 minutes. Rinse them well, pat dry and set aside.*

2 *Heat dry wok or skillet, add oil and sauté the leeks and turnips together until they are almost soft. Add the wine to the wok and simmer the vegetables, uncovered, for 5-10 minutes while the wine reduces and is absorbed into the vegetables.*

3 *Break up the tofu into a bowl. Beat in the spinach, onions, mushrooms, seeds and sea salt. Knead the mixture well until it binds together. Shape the tofu into round logs which are as long as the fish fillets are wide. Add a few T of arrowroot flour if the logs do not bind.*

4 *Heat oil in a wok or pan to deep frying temperature (180°-190°C) — see page 128 for deep-frying method. Deep fry the tofu logs until they are just set – do not cook them completely. Drain well on a rack or absorbent paper.*

5 *Roll each fish fillet around a tofu log and secure with toothpicks.*

6 *Smooth the vegetable mixture over the bottom of an oiled baking dish and place the fish rolls in one layer on top. Cover the dish and bake in 190°C oven for 10-15 minutes or until the fillets are cooked through.*

7 *Garnish with fresh coriander leaves.*

SWEET AND SOUR MARINADE FOR TOFU

(makes one cup)

¼ CUP RICE MISO

½ CUP BROWN RICE MALT SYRUP OR MALTOSE

½ CUP WATER OR STOCK

2-3 T BROWN RICE VINEGAR OR APPLE CIDER VINEGAR

2-3 T TOASTED SESAME OIL TO TASTE

2 T MINCED SHALLOTS, ONIONS OR RADISH

EXTRA *SHOYU* OR *TAMARI* AS NEEDED

1 *Place all ingredients in a processor and blend till smooth and creamy.*

2 *Cut the tofu into thin slices and prick it all over with a fork.*

3 *Marinate the tofu by pouring the marinade over the tofu.*

4 *Set it aside for several hours or overnight for best flavour.*

5 *Pour off the marinade and reserve it for the fillets.*

6 *If using for the fillets, dissolve 1 t of kuzu in a few teaspoons of cold water.*

7 *Combine marinade and dissolved kuzu in a saucepan and bring to the boil*

W	I	N	T	E	R

stirring continuously.

8 When thickened and boiled, serve over fillets, garnished with sprouts or minced parsley.

BROCCOLI WITH BLACK BEAN SAUCE

500 g BROCCOLI
1 T FERMENTED BLACK BEANS
3 T OIL
2 CLOVES FINELY CHOPPED GARLIC
2 T FINELY CHOPPED PEELED GINGER ROOT
2 t MAPLE SYRUP
SEA SALT TO TASTE
½ CUP STOCK OR WATER
1 t GROUND *KUZU* OR ARROWROOT
1 t ROASTED SESAME OIL
BLANCHED CARROT FLOWERS FOR GARNISH

1 Separate the broccoli head into bite-size florets. Peel the stems and slice thinly on the diagonal.

2 Rinse the black beans in water several times and shake dry. Chop coarsely.

3 Heat dry wok or skillet, add oil and briefly sauté the black beans, garlic and ginger root. Add the broccoli stalks and sauté quickly. Lower heat, add broccoli florets and sauté until they change colour.

4 Add maple syrup, sea salt and stock or water. Cover wok and simmer 2-3 minutes.

5 Dissolve kuzu in 2 T cold water. Add to the broccoli and sauté until the sauce thickens.

6 To serve, season with roasted sesame oil and garnish with carrot flowers.

M A C R O B I O T I C S & B E Y O N D

Winter Menu 3: Broccoli Cauliflower Mousseline
Spiced Chickpeas with Mochi Topping
Snow Pea Arame Salad

BROCCOLI CAULIFLOWER MOUSSELINE

4 EGGS

1 ¼ CUPS GROUND LIGHTLY TOASTED ALMONDS

½ CUP PLAIN YOGHURT

SEA SALT AND FRESHLY GROUND PEPPER TO TASTE

3 CUPS COOKED BROCCOLI FLORETS

3 CUPS COOKED CAULIFLOWER FLORETS

Lemon *Tamari* Sauce

2 T GROUND *KUZU* OR ARROWROOT

2½ CUPS WATER

2-3 T *TAMARI* TO TASTE

1 T LEMON JUICE

1 t FRESHLY GRATED GINGER JUICE (see p. 127)

Forward planning: *You will need steaming equipment, such as a wok and bamboo steaming basket, to hold the mousseline moulds. Oil 8-10 ½-cup moulds or oriental teacups.*

1 *Beat the eggs and combine with the almonds, yoghurt and seasonings.*

2 *Purée the broccoli with half of the egg mixture, and purée the cauliflower with the other half.*

3 *Fill the oiled moulds three-quarters full, alternating the broccoli and cauliflower purées. Create a layered or marbled effect as you choose.*

4 *Fold a piece of oiled aluminium foil over each mould, taking care that it does not touch the mousseline.*

5 *Put the moulds into the steamer. Put a lid on the steamer and steam for 15 minutes or until the mousseline is almost set. Ceramic moulds will be slower than glass or metal moulds.*

6 *Serve in the moulds with heated Lemon Tamari Sauce.*

7 *Dissolve the kuzu in a small amount of the cold water, in a saucepan. Add the remaining water and tamari.*

8 *Bring to the boil, stirring continuously. Remove from the stove and add the lemon and ginger juices.*

W   I   N   T   E   R

SPICED CHICKPEAS WITH MOCHI TOPPING

2 CUPS DRY CHICKPEAS, SOAKED OVERNIGHT IN WATER (COVER BY AT LEAST 5 cm)
2 t CUMIN SEEDS
3 T OIL
1 CUP FINELY CHOPPED ONION
2 T FINELY CHOPPED GARLIC
2 T FINELY CHOPPED GINGER ROOT
2 t GROUND CUMIN
1½ t GROUND TURMERIC
1 t GROUND CORIANDER
½ t GROUND CARDAMON
½ t GROUND CLOVES
½ t GROUND CINNAMON
¼ t GROUND BLACK PEPPER
CHILI PEPPER TO TASTE

Topping

⅓ CUP MISO
⅔ CUP TAHINI
3 PIECES GRATED MOCHI
SLIVERED SHALLOTS OR PARSLEY FOR GARNISH

Forward planning: *The chickpeas may be cooked with the spices the night or morning before serving. Preheat oven to 200°C. Reserve chickpea cooking liquid for Menu 4.*

1   Drain chickpeas and discard soaking water. Cover peas by at least 3 cm with fresh water and bring to the boil. Simmer for 20 minutes uncovered, skimming off residue that rises to the top.

2   Add more water if necessary. Cover the pot and cook the peas for about 2 more hours until they are soft. Alternatively, pressure cook them for about one hour.

3   Drain the chickpeas and reserve the cooking liquid.

4   Toast cumin seeds to increase their flavour. Be careful not to burn them.

5   Heat dry skillet, add oil and sauté the cumin seeds and onion until the onion is soft and transparent. Add the garlic and ginger root and all the spices. Sauté the mixture until the spices are well absorbed and have released their flavour.

6   Stir the chickpeas and 1 cup of reserved chickpea cooking liquid into the spice mixture. Bring to a soft boil, cover the pot and gently simmer for 30 minutes, stirring occasionally. Watch that the mixture does not stick and begin to burn, and add more cooking liquid if necessary.

7   To make Mochi Topping: Cream the miso *and tahini together with a little boiling water. Mix the grated* mochi *into the* miso *tahini sauce.*

8   Put the chickpeas into an ovenproof dish and spread the Mochi *Topping over them. Cover the dish. Bake in a 200°C oven for 15-20 minutes until the topping is smooth.*

9   Uncover the dish and brown the topping lightly in the oven.

10 Garnish with slivered shallots or parsley.

SNOW PEA ARAME SALAD

¾ CUP DRIED *ARAME*

2 CUPS SNOW PEAS, STRINGED AND CUT IN TWO ON THE DIAGONAL

½ CUP ROASTED SUNFLOWER SEEDS

Vinaigrette Dressing

1–2 GARLIC CLOVES

2 T OLIVE OIL

1 EGG

SEA SALT

1 T PREPARED MUSTARD

½ –1 t JAPANESE LEMON PEPPER OR FRESHLY GROUND BLACK PEPPER

2 T BROWN RICE VINEGAR

¼ CUP OLIVE OIL

Forward planning: *The Dressing may be prepared one or more days in advance.*

Dressing

1   Put the sea salt on a paper bag and crush the garlic into it with the flat blade of a knife until it is pasty. Whisk the garlic with the 2 T olive oil, egg, mustard and pepper, and gradually beat in the vinegar.

2   Add the ¼-⅓ cup olive oil in a thin stream, whisking until the dressing is smooth and creamy.

Salad

3   Wash the arame *well and soak in water to cover for 3 minutes.*

4   Place the snow peas in a strainer and immerse in boiling salted water for no more than 1 minute. Drain immediately and rinse quickly under cold water to stop further cooking. They must be green and crisp. Shake dry.

5   Drain arame *and drop into the boiling water and boil for 5 minutes. Drain and rinse under cold water. Shake dry.*

6   Gently combine the arame *and snow peas in a salad bowl. Pour the dressing over the salad and toss with the sunflower seeds.*

W	I	N	T	E	R

Winter Menu 4: Split Pea Soup
Carrots in Orange Juice
Buckwheat with Fennel, Onions and Mush-
rooms

SPLIT PEA SOUP

2 CUPS DRY SPLIT PEAS
6 CUPS WATER
1 BAY LEAF
1 LARGE RED CAPSICUM/PEPPER
1 CUP DICED ONIONS
½ CUP CHOPPED CELERY
SEA SALT, *SHOYO* OR *MISO* TO TASTE
CHOPPED PARSLEY FOR GARNISH
MINCED ANCHOVIES (OR OLIVES IF FOLLOWING A VEGAN DIET) FOR GARNISH

Forward planning: *Prepare capsicum the night before. Soak peas overnight.*
1   Wash split peas quickly and drain them.
2   Add the split peas to the 6 cups of water in a saucepan and bring to the boil. Lower the heat and simmer, uncovered, for 30 minutes, skimming off residue that rises to the top.
3   Put in the bay leaf. Add more water if too much has evaporated, cover the pan and simmer for another 30 minutes. Alternatively, pressure cook for 15 minutes.
4   While the peas are cooking, prepare the capsicum. Using a fork to hold it, rotate the capsicum over a gas flame or electric hotplate until the skin is charred. Alternatively, bake it in a 200°C oven for about 10 minutes. Place the capsicum in a paper bag until it is cool enough to handle, and then peel under running water. Remove seeds. Chop the capsicum finely.
5   Uncover pan and add the onions and celery. Cover and simmer for another 10 minutes. Add more water if the soup is too thick, until the desired thickness is obtained.
6   Remove bay leaf. Add the capsicum. Add seasoning to taste. Cover and simmer another few minutes.
7   To serve, garnish with chopped parsley and minced anchovies or olives.

CARROTS IN ORANGE JUICE

8 CUPS SHREDDED CARROTS

4 T OIL

GRATED RIND AND JUICE OF 1 LARGE ORANGE

SEA SALT AND FRESHLY GROUND PEPPER TO TASTE

1 T MINCED FRESH CORIANDER LEAVES FOR GARNISH

1   Heat dry wok or skillet pan. Add the oil and quickly sauté the carrots and grated orange rind over high heat for 2 minutes.

2   Add the orange juice and continue to sauté the carrots for another 2 minutes over high heat while the orange juice reduces.

3   Season with sea salt and pepper to taste. Reduce heat and cook for several minutes more until the carrots are almost soft.

4   Place carrots on a serving dish. Reduce the liquid to 1 T. Pour over the carrots.

5   To serve, garnish with fresh minced coriander leaves.

BUCKWHEAT WITH FENNEL, ONIONS AND MUSHROOMS

¾ CUP ROASTED BUCKWHEAT GROATS

1 EGG

1 CUP WATER

6 T OIL

2 CUPS THINLY SLICED ONION RINGS

3 CUPS SLICED MUSHROOMS

3 CUPS THINLY SLICED FENNEL BULBS

SEA SALT

JAPANESE LEMON PEPPER OR FRESHLY GROUND BLACK PEPPER TO TASTE

1 CUP PINE NUTS

EXTRA OIL AS NEEDED

Forward planning: *Buckwheat may be prepared 1 day in advance (see steps 1-3 below).*

1   Beat the egg and stir through the buckwheat groats to coat each grain. Put the buckwheat into a heavy saucepan.

2   Pour 1 cup of water over the grains, add a pinch of sea salt, and bring to the boil. Lower heat, cover pan and simmer gently for 15 minutes or until the buckwheat is cooked.

3   Pack the cooked buckwheat into an oiled loaf pan or mould and leave to cool.

4   Heat dry wok or skillet, add 2 T of oil and sauté the onions until they are transparent. Add the mushrooms and cook until they are soft. Season with sea salt

W	I	N	T	E	R

and pepper to taste.

5   Heat dry wok or skillet, add another 2 T of oil and sauté the fennel until it is golden brown and almost soft. Add sea salt and pepper to taste when the fennel has begun to soften.

6   Turn the buckwheat out of the mould and cut into slices. Heat dry skillet, add the remaining oil and sauté the pine nuts until lightly browned. Remove from skillet.

7   Sauté buckwheat slices, adding more oil as needed, until slices are warm (optional).

8   To serve, combine the vegetables and pine nuts and decorate the buckwheat slices with them on each plate.

Winter Menu 5:   Layered Vegetable Casserole
Endive, Radish and Mandarin Salad

LAYERED VEGETABLE CASSEROLE

SHEETS OF TOASTED *NORI*

3 CUPS THINLY SLICED ONION RINGS

2 CUPS THINLY SLICED SWEET POTATO CIRCLES

GROUND *KUZU* OR ARROWROOT (FOR THICKENING SAUCE)

MINCED FRESH CORIANDER LEAVES FOR GARNISH

Sauce

4 T TAHINI OR ROASTED ALMOND BUTTER

¾ T *MISO* (*NATTO MISO* IS GOOD FOR THIS DISH)

3 MASHED *UMEBOSHI* PLUMS OR 1 T *UMEBOSHI* PASTE,
   OR 3 T BROWN RICE VINEGAR

1-2 T *TAMARI* OR *SHOYO*

½ CUP *MIRIN*

Forward planning: *Sauce can be made in advance. Preheat oven to 190°C.*

1   Blend the five Sauce ingredients together.

2   Toast nori sheets by moving them, shiny side down, back and forth at least 5 cm above a low gas or electric flame until they are green when you hold them up to the light.

3   Cover the base of an oiled casserole with a single layer of nori.

4   Cover the nori with a layer of onion rings and a layer of sweet potato circles.

5   Spoon some of the Sauce over the vegetables.

6 Continue layering with nori, onions, sweet potato and Sauce, using all of these ingredients and ending with the Sauce.

7 Cover the casserole and bake in preheated oven for 45-60 minutes or until the vegetables are soft.

8 If cooking liquid remains, strain it carefully from the casserole into a small saucepan. Dissolve 1-2 t kuzu per cup of liquid in cold water. Add to the liquid and bring to the boil, stirring continuously. Spoon over the vegetables.

9 To serve, garnish with minced fresh coriander leaves.

ENDIVE, RADISH and MANDARIN SALAD

1 HEAD CURLY ENDIVE
1 CUP THINLY SLICED RADISHES
2 MANDARINS SEPARATED INTO SECTIONS
ALFALFA SPROUTS AND PITTED OLIVES FOR GARNISH
Tofu dressing
300 g TOFU
1 CUP FINELY MINCED FRESH PARSLEY LEAVES
¼ CUP BROWN RICE VINEGAR
2 t PREPARED MUSTARD
SEA SALT TO TASTE
JAPANESE LEMON PEPPER OR FRESHLY GROUND BLACK PEPPER TO TASTE
¼ CUP OIL

Forward planning: *Dressing should be made at least one day in advance, to develop flavour. Keep uncovered in refrigerator. Stir and thin with hot liquid to desired consistency when ready to use.*

Dressing

1 Blanch tofu by dropping into boiling water for 1 minute and draining it well.

2 Break the tofu into chunks and blend with the parsley, vinegar, mustard, salt and pepper until the mixture is smooth and creamy. Add the oil slowly in a thin stream and blend until the mixture is well emulsified.

Salad

3 Separate the head of endive, trimming coarse stems. Arrange the endive stalks in a spoke pattern on a plate. Arrange the radishes in a circle in the middle of the plate and cover with a smaller circle of mandarin sections.

4 Spoon Dressing over the salad.

5 Garnish with sprouts and olives.

SPRING

Spring is Nature's birthing season, a time of development and creation where life is re-awakened after the long dark winter. We all feel this — a sense of energy wanting to 'spring' forth and blossom into what's to come. You may feel a new burst of inspiration, power and sparkle, and be almost unable to contain yourself any longer. You will notice the young sprouts and shoots of spring just pushing their way up through the cold earth: they too are bursting forth from confinement.

It's a time for planting and planning: gardens, relationships, work, play, study — all at our finger tips and all we have to do is make the most of them.

Because growth is such a vital part of spring, the element associated with this season is Wood, which reflects the rhythms of life in trees and plants. This element governs the liver and gall bladder, and an imbalance in this element can result in such problems as poor flexibility or a weakness in the root system of an individual (as in roots of a tree).

The most logical colour association with spring is naturally green — the fresh and wholesome green of young plants. It is believed that someone who is either particularly attracted to green or really avoids green like the plague may have his or her Wood element out of balance. Sometimes a greenish tinge appears on the skin of the face, especially in the cheeks and around the eyes, if this is the case.

The Wood element is said to be responsible for our mental clarity or lack of it, and our ability to focus, plan and make decisions. When poor judgement becomes apparent, and planning and organisation are neglected, then a Wood imbalance is likely to be the cause. On the other hand, you may find that you are increasingly preoccupied with making decisions, and trying to organise everything and everyone. If you are in this frame of mind you may have a hard time letting go and just relaxing, and you could possibly suffer from tension in the back, neck, shoulders and head areas.

Suppressed anger can most certainly injure the Wood element, or more specifically the liver and gall bladder; generally speaking, any suppressed emotion does not allow you to balance your energy, and could lead to more serious problems.

The liver is important because it is responsible for storing and distributing nourishment for the entire body; it is involved both with the formation and breakdown of blood and in filtering toxins from the blood (toxins being unusable materials that need to be eliminated from the body to keep balance and order). The liver cells make bile which aids in digestion and is retained in the gall bladder so that it can be used in the intestines for the breakdown and absorption of fats. Bile also aids the metabolism of proteins and carbohydrates, helping to regulate the blood-

MACROBIOTICS & BEYOND

sugar level by changing proteins and fats into glucose, a simple sugar that is used by all the cells.

Each spring we are given a new opportunity to renew our arrangements for our internal and external settings. This includes assessing how to nourish ourselves with the body's fuel — *food!* Most of us are now conscious that the *way* that we choose to eat, *what* we choose to eat, *how much* we choose to eat and *when* we choose to eat it, are all significant factors in maintaining health and vitality. Not eating when we are upset, in a hurry, or tense, is actually wise as the body cannot deal with too much all at once. We should take only what we need, when we need it, and take the time to chew and digest our foods, without rushing around.

Wholefoods are more nourishing and satisfying than refined foods as they have more vital life force for us to use. In the spring many of us are aware that there is a desire to cleanse both internally and externally, and this can be done by abstaining from foods for a while, by choosing one food on which to 'fast' or by simple eating less. Some people like to start off in spring by going on a raw foods/fruit juice diet for a few days — this relieves the digestive organs of excessive amounts of fats which have been taken in during the wintertime to keep ourselves warmer. The liver, too, can be assisted by this type of diet, as it can relieve itself of toxins accumulated in the previous season. Remember, however, that fasting is not for everyone, especially if you have a low body temperature most of the time. Fasting can lower your body temperature even further and although it may achieve one thing it can set other organs out of balance. So be sure to check before choosing how you will cleanse yourself.

You can test to see which specific foods are related to your symptoms. In the first seven to ten days, eliminate various foods such as those containing caffeine, alcohol, dairy products, seeds, nuts and grains, and eat only fresh vegetables for three days. Then switch to freshly made juices for two days and follow with a further two days of water only. Now, over the next seven days slowly begin to introduce one food at a time back into your diet, noting what each one does for you, and how you feel. Keep alternating your vegetables, fruits and grains, and see how comfortable you feel, and what happens.

If you feel you are a 'cold' type, then the best foods for the first four days will be vegetable broths as opposed to raw vegetable juices. During this time, it would be a good idea to choose some other cleansing therapies, such as massage and sauna baths — a good sweat always helps to cleanse the blood. Whatever avenue you choose, I'm sure that you will find the one that works best for you!

Spring is the perfect time to be open, nourished and sensitive both to your needs and the needs of others. So, take the time to clean out the past to make room for the new. Be aware of the opportunities that are presented to you, and take advantage of all that is available — choosing the most appropriate way for you to be fulfilled.

S　　P　　R　　I　　N　　G

Spring Menus

1　Buddha's Casserole
　Mustard Pickles

2　Basil Chicken
　Walnut Vegetable Salad

3　Spring Fish Tarts
　Eggplant Orientale

4　Dilled Leek and Zucchini Soup or Almond Potato Puffs
　Bean Salad

5　Apricot Leek Crepes
　Broad Bean Salad

NOTE: The menus in this book serve 4 – 6 people.

Spring Menu 1:　Buddha's Casserole
　　　　　　　　　Mustard Pickles

BUDDHA'S CASSEROLE

LETTUCE LEAVES

12 DRIED CHINESE BLACK MUSHROOMS, SOAKED 4 HOURS IN AT LEAST 1 CUP COLD WATER

8 CLOUD EAR MUSHROOMS, SOAKED 1 HOUR IN COLD WATER

15 DRIED LOTUS SEEDS, SOAKED IN COLD WATER OVERNIGHT

½ CUP DRIED CHESTNUTS, SOAKED IN COLD WATER OVERNIGHT

1 kg THINLY SLICED *SEITAN* GLUTEN MEAT * (SEE GLOSSARY)

500 g FIRM 2.5 cm TOFU CUBES (TOSSED IN ARROWROOT)

1 CUP SLICED FRESH BAMBOO SHOOTS

250 g STRINGED SNOW PEAS

ROASTED SESAME OIL

Braising Liquid

4 T *SHOYU* OR *TAMARI*

6 T WHITE WINE

2 t MAPLE SYRUP

1 CUP STOCK
1 CUP MUSHROOM SOAKING LIQUID

Forward planning: *Soak lotus seeds and chestnuts overnight.*

1   Line large fireproof casserole with lettuce leaves.

2   Drain black mushrooms and reserve 1 cup of soaking liquid. Discard stems and cut caps into quarters.

3   Drain cloud ears, lotus seeds and chestnuts and discard liquid.

4   Heat oil in wok or pan to deep frying temperature (180° – 190°C) – see page 128 for deep frying method. Without overcrowding the pan, deep-fry seitan slices in batches for a few minutes, only until sealed (indicated by the outside bubbling slightly). Drain slices well and rinse under cold running water to remove excess oil.

5   Deep fry, drain and rinse tofu cubes in the same manner. Dry cubes well.

6   Place all ingredients except tofu cubes and snow peas in the lined casserole.

7   Combine Braising Liquid ingredients and spoon over the casserole. Bring casserole to the boil, cover and lower heat to simmering. Test vegetables after 25 minutes. If soft, add tofu and snow peas and simmer another 5 minutes. Otherwise, test every 5 minutes and add tofu and snow peas for the last 5 minutes.

8   To serve, sprinkle roasted sesame oil over the casserole. Serve over rice or noodles. Accompany with mustard pickles.

MUSTARD PICKLES

3 – 4 LEBANESE (SHORT, SMOOTH-SKINNED) CUCUMBERS
2 T BROWN RICE VINEGAR
2 – 3 T BROWN RICE MALT SYRUP OR BARLEY MALT
1 t OIL
1 T COARSE—GRAIN PREPARED MUSTARD
1 t SEA SALT

1   Slice cucumbers crosswise thinly and place in a jar.

2   Combine remaining ingredients in a saucepan and heat until warm.

3   Pour marinade over cucumber slices. Pickles will keep several weeks if refrigerated.

S P R I N G

Spring Menu 2: Basil Chicken
Cooked Vegetable Salad and
Walnut Vinaigrette

BASIL CHICKEN

Chicken

4 CUPS CHICKEN STOCK

¼ CUP FRESH LIME JUICE

125 g FRESH BASIL LEAVES

FRESHLY GROUND BLACK PEPPER TO TASTE

2 OR 3 375 g CHICKEN BREASTS, SKINNED, BONED, TRIMMED AND HALVED

Spring Mayonnaise

300 g TOFU

1 T MINCED SHALLOTS

2 T LEMON JUICE

2 t COARSE—GRAIN PREPARED MUSTARD

¼ CUP OLIVE OIL

½ CUP SESAME OR OTHER OIL

2 T MINCED FRESH TARRAGON; ALTERNATIVELY, 1 T MINCED FRESH PARSLEY
PLUS 1 t MINCED FRESH THYME

SEA SALT

Sesame Ginger Toasts

½ CUP SESAME OR OLIVE OIL

1 t ROASTED SESAME OIL

1 t GROUND GINGER SPICE

1 MINCED GARLIC CLOVE

1 LOAF WHOLEWHEAT FRENCH OR ITALIAN BREAD, CUT CROSSWISE INTO 1 cm
THICK SLICES

Forward planning: *Mayonnaise may be prepared in advance — ideally, at least one day in advance, so that its flavour has time to develop. Keep it uncovered in the refrigerator. Stir and thin with hot liquid to desired consistency when ready to use. Chicken must be cooked one day in advance. Preheat oven to 200°C.*

Chicken

1 Combine stock, lime juice, basil and pepper in a pan large enough to hold the chicken breasts in one layer. Bring to the boil.

2 Place breasts in liquid without overlapping, cover and simmer 3 – 4 minutes.

3 Remove pan from heat and set aside until cooled to room temperature.

4 Transfer contents to a bowl. Cover and leave overnight.

Spring Mayonnaise

5 Blanch tofu by dropping into boiling water for 1 minute. Drain well.

6 Break tofu into chunks and blend with shallots, lemon juice and mustard until the mixture is smooth and creamy. Add the oil slowly in a thin stream and blend until thick.

7 Stir in herbs and sea salt to taste.

Sesame Ginger Toasts

8 Combine oils, ginger and garlic and heat in a small saucepan until warm. Remove from heat.

9 Brush both sides of bread slices with oil mixture.

10 Arrange slices on baking sheets and bake 10 minutes or until golden.

To serve:

11 Remove chicken breasts from liquid and slice thinly.

12 Arrange chicken slices in the middle of a serving plate and surround with Ginger Toasts. Serve Mayonnaise separately.

WALNUT VEGETABLE SALAD

250 g FRESH ASPARAGUS STALKS
2½ CUPS 3 cm LENGTH GREEN BEANS, STRINGLESS IF POSSIBLE
2½ CUPS 3 cm MATCHSTICKS CARROTS
2½ CUPS 1 cm THICK ROUNDS ZUCCHINI, 2.5 cm IN DIAMETER
Dressing
¼ CUP VINEGAR
SEA SALT AND FRESHLY GROUND BLACK PEPPER TO TASTE
¾ CUP WALNUT OIL
½ CUP FINELY GROUND WALNUTS

Forward planning: *Dressing should be prepared several hours in advance.*

Vegetables

1 Peel bottom 5 cm of asparagus stalks and cut stalks into 3 cm lengths.

2 Cook vegetables in separate batches in boiling water until tender. Refresh each batch under running cold water and drain well.

Dressing

3 Blend vinegar with sea salt and pepper to taste.

4 Blend in oil slowly in a thin stream until dressing is well emulsified. Add ground walnuts.

To serve:

5 Toss vegetables with the Dressing.

S   P   R   I   N   G

Spring Menu 3:   Spring Fish Tarts
Eggplant Orientale

SPRING FISH TARTS

Pastry

550 g GROUND WHITE FLESH FISH (E.G. SNAPPER, REDFISH, BREAM)

1 – 2 T GROUND *KUZU* OR ARROWROOT

1½ t DRIED BASIL

1¼ t DRIED THYME

1 t DRIED OREGANO

½ t GARLIC POWDER

½ t GROUND CORIANDER

SEA SALT AND JAPANESE CHILI POWDER

1 EGG WHITE (OPTIONAL)

Vegetable Filling

1 T OIL

1½ CUPS MINCED SHALLOTS OR SPRING ONIONS

1 t CUMIN SEED

1½ CUPS DICED ZUCCHINI

1 CUP CHOPPED CHINESE CABBAGE OR BEAN SPROUTS

SEA SALT AND FRESHLY GROUND BLACK PEPPER

Tofu Nut Cream

600 g TOFU

1 CUP GROUND NUTS

½ CUP SOY MAYONNAISE, ALMOND OR CASHEW NUT BUTTER, OR OIL

½ CUP CAPERS OR FINELY CHOPPED PICKLES (GINGER, OLIVES, *DAIKON*)

BLANCHED VEGETABLES FOR GARNISH, E.G. BROCCOLI OR CARROT FLOWERS

Forward planning: *Preheat oven to 180°C.*

Pastry

1   Combine all pastry ingredients together well.

2   Press fish pastry into individual tart forms. Brush with egg white if desired.

3   Bake in 180°C oven for 12 – 15 minutes.

Vegetable Filling

4   Heat wok or skillet, add oil and sauté shallots or spring onions with the cumin seed until transparent.

5   Add zucchini and cabbage or bean sprouts and sea salt and pepper to taste. Cover and simmer until the vegetables are almost soft.

Tofu Nut Cream

6 Blanch tofu by dropping into boiling water for 1 minute and draining well.

7 Break tofu into chunks and blend well with remaining ingredients.

To serve:

8 Either stir vegetables into tofu cream and fill pastry, or place vegetables into tarts and cover with tofu cream.

9 Warm tarts in the oven for a few minutes. Decorate with cut blanched vegetables.

EGGPLANT ORIENTALE

1 EGGPLANT, NOT MORE THAN 7.5 cm IN DIAMETER
OIL AS NEEDED, AT LEAST 3 – 4 T
2 T *MIRIN*
LETTUCE LEAVES
1 T TOASTED SESAME SEEDS FOR GARNISH
Sauce
⅓ CUP WHITE RICE *MISO*
½ EGG YOLK
2 T *MIRIN*
1 T STOCK
1 t MAPLE SYRUP (OPTIONAL)
1 t FINELY GRATED LEMON RIND

1 Blend Sauce ingredients in small saucepan or double boiler, stirring continuously over medium heat with wooden spoon until sauce thickens and is creamy. Do not boil. Remove from heat.

2 Cut eggplant into 1 cm thick slices and pat dry.

3 Heat skillet, add oil and sauté eggplant slices for 3 –4 minutes on each side.

4 With skillet lid ready to prevent splattering, add mirin and cover pan quickly. Cook a further 2 – 3 minutes or until soft.

5 To serve, place eggplant slices on lettuce leaves, spoon sauce over and garnish with sesame seeds.

NOTE: This recipe can be made with other vegetables, e.g. squash, zucchini, blanched spinach or cauliflower.

S   P   R   I   N   G

Spring Menu 4: Dilled Leek and Zucchini Soup
or Almond Potato Puffs
Bean Salad

DILLED LEEK AND ZUCCHINI SOUP

¼ CUP OIL

3 CUPS CHOPPED LEEKS

4 CUPS CHOPPED ZUCCHINI

⅛ CUP SNIPPED FRESH DILL

1 t DILL SEEDS

SEA SALT AND FRESHLY GROUND BLACK PEPPER

5 CUPS STOCK

MINCED PARSLEY OR SHALLOTS FOR GARNISH

1   *Heat skillet, add oil and sauté leeks until transparent.*
2   *Add zucchini and sauté until soft.*
3   *Add dill, dill seeds and sea salt and freshly ground pepper to taste.*
4   *Stir in stock, bring to the boil and simmer, partially covered, for 15 minutes. Remove from heat and allow to cool slightly.*
5   *Purée or blend half the soup and return to the pot.*
6   *To serve, reheat soup and garnish with minced parsley or shallots.*

ALMOND POTATO PUFFS

¼ CUP WATER OR STOCK

2 T OIL

3 T WHOLEWHEAT FLOUR

1 EGG

1½ CUPS COOKED MASHED NEW POTATOES

SEA SALT

½ CUP BLANCHED FINELY CHOPPED ALMONDS

OIL FOR DEEP-FRYING

1   *Combine water or stock and oil in a small saucepan and bring to the boil.*
2   *Remove immediately from the heat, add flour all at once and beat until mixture is smooth. Beat in the egg. Set aside to cool.*
3   *When cool, add mashed potatoes and sea salt (to taste) to flour-egg mixture and blend well.*
4   *Flour hands with arrowroot flour and shape mixture into balls the size of walnuts in the shell. Dip balls into cold water and roll in the chopped almonds.*

MACROBIOTICS & BEYOND

5   Heat oil in a wok or pan to deep-frying temperature (180° – 190°C) — See page 128 for deep-frying method. Deep fry puffs until golden brown. Drain well.
6   Serve with mustard.

BEAN SALAD

1 CUP DRIED KIDNEY OR BARLOTTI BEANS, SOAKED OVERNIGHT IN WATER TO COVER BY AT LEAST 5 cm
½ CUP DRIED CHICKPEAS, SOAKED OVERNIGHT IN WATER TO COVER BY AT LEAST 5 cm
2 PIECES *KOMBU* (OPTIONAL)
2 BAY LEAVES
2 CUPS FRESH GREEN BEANS
***Miso* Dressing**
½ CUP *MISO*
1 CUP GROUND MACADAMIA NUTS
1 CUP OIL
1 CUP MINCED ONION
¼ CUP MINCED CELERY
¼ CUP MINCED PARSLEY
¼ CUP GRATED CARROT
¼ CUP GRATED ZUCCHINI
¼ CUP MINCED PICKLES (OLIVES, *DAIKON*, GINGER)

Forward planning: Soak beans and chickpeas separately overnight. Blanch beans. Prepare dressing.

1   Drain beans and chickpeas. Add fresh water to cover the beans and chickpeas by at least 3 cm in separate pots. Bring to the boil, lower heat and simmer, uncovered, for 30 minutes, skimming off residue that rises to the top. Add more water if necessary.

2   Add kombu and bay leaf to each pot. Cover and boil until beans and chickpeas are just soft. Do not overcook or they will fall apart.

3   While beans and chickpeas are cooking, blanch whole greens beans in boiling water. Refresh under cold running water, drain and slice thinly. Reserve until serving salad.

4   Also while beans are cooking, prepare miso Dressing. Blend miso, nuts and oil, adding a few drops of hot water if necessary, until the mixture is creamy. Stir in the remaining ingredients.

5   When beans and chickpeas are cooked, drain and combine them with miso

SPRING

Dressing while still hot. Allow to sit for at least 2 – 3 hours before serving.
6   Just before serving, toss with the sliced green beans.

Spring Menu 5:   Apricot Leek Crepes
Broad Bean Salad

APRICOT LEEK CREPES

Crepes

3 EGGS

⅔ CUP BUCKWHEAT OR WHOLEWHEAT FLOUR

½ t SEA SALT

1 CUP SOYMILK OR ALMOND MILK (see tofu loaf recipe on page 55)

Filling

½ CUP COUSCOUS

¾ CUP BOILING WATER OR STOCK

6 T OIL

1 CUP FINELY CHOPPED ONION

2 LARGE LEEKS, WASHED, TRIMMED AND FINELY CHOPPED

¾ CUP UNSULPHURED APRICOTS, SOAKED OVERNIGHT IN BOILING WATER, PITTED AND FINELY CHOPPED

1 CUP MINCED WHITE FLESHED FISH

2 T FINELY CHOPPED PARSLEY

2–3 t FINELY CHOPPED MINT (OR TO TASTE)

½ t CINNAMON OR GROUND CORIANDER

SEA SALT

Green Sauce

8 CUPS LIGHTLY PACKED CHOPPED SPINACH LEAVES

3 CUPS LIGHTLY PACKED FRESH PARSLEY LEAVES

1 PEELED GARLIC CLOVE

3 x 7 cm STEMMED THYME OR OREGANO SPRIGS

½ t OIL

2 T LEMON JUICE

FRESHLY GROUND BLACK PEPPER TO TASTE

SEA SALT TO TASTE

2 T OIL

MACROBIOTICS & BEYOND

Forward planning: *Green Sauce may be made in advance and stored in a glass jar in the refrigerator. Soak apricots overnight. Preheat oven to 180°C.*

Crepes

1   *Combine crepe ingredients and beat to a smooth batter. Let stand for 30 minutes.*

2   *For each crepe, pour 2 T batter into heated oiled 17 cm crepe pan or skillet. Cook crepe on one side only, until lightly browned.*

3   *Remove and press, cooked side down, into large oiled muffin tins or small oiled soufflé dishes.*

Filling

4   *Pour boiling water or stock over couscous and set aside for 10 minutes.*

5   *Heat skillet, add oil and sauté onions until transparent. Add leeks, cover skillet and cook until soft.*

6   *Add apricots, fish, herbs and spice, and sea salt to taste. Cook until the fish is tender.*

7   *Remove all but 2 – 3 T of liquid. Fold in couscous.*

Green Sauce

8   *Mince spinach and parsley finely together. Crush garlic by putting sea salt on a paper bag and crushing garlic into it with the flat blade of a knife until it is pasty. Combine spinach and parsley with crushed garlic, herbs, lemon juice, ½ t oil, sea salt and pepper, and blend until the mixture is smooth and creamy.*

9   *Slowly drip in the remaining 2 T oil and blend until oil is absorbed.*

To complete dish:

10 *Fill crepes three-quarters full with apricot leek mixture. Place in 180°C oven and cook for 15 minutes.*

11 *Spoon Green Sauce over mixture and cook for another 15 minutes or until filling is set.*

NOTE: Use leftover Green Sauce with fish, vegetables, grains or beans.

BROAD BEAN SALAD

500 g BROAD BEANS IN THEIR PODS
ROASTED SESAME SEEDS FOR GARNISH

Vinegar Dressing

2 T BROWN RICE VINEGAR
2 T *SHOYU* OR *TAMARI*
2 T STOCK
1 – 2 CLOVES PEELED CRUSHED GARLIC (see green sauce section of apricot

SPRING

leek crepes, page 45)

4 T CHOPPED PARSLEY

2 T OIL

½ – 1 T *MISO* OR SEA SALT

1 Drop beans (in pods) into boiling salted water, cover and cook until tender.
2 Drain and shell beans.
3 Blend Vinegar Dressing ingredients.
4 Pour Dressing over beans and marinate 2 – 3 hours.
5 Before serving, drain off any excess Dressing and sprinkle with roasted sesame seeds.

SUMMER

Summer is Nature's season of maturation and growth. All the colourful flowers, fruits and vegetables blossom into existence, along with a personal feeling of energy and vitality. An abundance of action and outward movement are positive aspects which can lead to increased travel, restlessness, and playing out in the sunshine.

The element Fire, which depicts and characterises summer, is noted for providing the energy governing the heart and small intestines. It is also associated with the organ known as 'Circulation-Sex' which is said to protect the heart and regulate blood flow, nourishment and heat throughout the body. The other system sometimes associated with the Fire element is called the 'Triple Heater' and it provides warmth and regulates body temperature.

The heart moves the blood and carries oxygen and other nutrients to the rest of the body. The small intestine, on the other hand, connects the stomach to the large intestine and is divided into three parts. Proper care and functioning of the small intestine is one of the keys to our nourishment because the only nutrients we can actually use are those which we assimilate and digest through it.

Of course other factors are relevant, such as how well we chew our food — especially cereal grains and breads — and how well our stomach is functioning. When the food is converted into a liquid state, with the help of the enzymes from the pancreas, bile from the gall bladder and liver, plus other substances, the small intestine transforms the foods we eat into useable components like amino acids, fatty acids and glucose. These are then absorbed into the bloodstream from the small intestines and transported to the liver, which will either distribute them for immediate use or store them in the form of glycogen until needed.

How we balance out the Fire element in the form of heat depends entirely upon our nature. Some of us may prefer a cool shower or swim, others may seek to wear the watery colour blue or be surrounded by blue colour. Blue balances red, which is the colour connected with Fire; they control each other by keeping each other in balance. Blue, associated with the kidney and bladder energy, is related to female energy, whereas Fire is related to male sexual energy and creative potential.

We generally need a diet which is cooling and light, and Nature has provided us with just the right fruits and vegetables to eat at this time of the year. Light cooking or a raw foods diet balance out the summer's heat, which in turn helps us feel lighter, keeps our weight down and keeps our energy up.

Fruits are the most cooling foods, followed by vegetables. The more concentrated foods like seeds, nuts, animal flesh, fats and complex carbohydrates have a heating aspect to them, and should be used in minimal quantities, if at all.

S	U	M	M	E	R

Fruit and vegetable juices, fish and seafood, lightly cooked vegetables and noodles support our energy and at the same time keep us feeling cool and refreshed.

Obviously, if you are very active outdoors or doing lots of physical exercise, then you need to eat more. Be sparing with fried foods and chips, processed and chemical foods, and drugs of any nature — especially caffeine and alcohol.

Leafy green vegetables with a bitter taste, like endive, lettuce, watercress and escarole, are good to include in your weekly diet. Remember, too much can also be harmful, so if the Fire element is too weak or too strong there may be a strong repulsion or attraction toward bitter-flavoured foods. For people with too much Fire, too much energy, who are too red in the face, who love to talk incessantly and socialise and laugh constantly, a cooling diet consisting primarily of shellfish, vegetables and fruits would be most suitable. However, weak Fire types need more wholegrains or noodles, fish, chicken, cooked vegetables and some hot spices which will add a little more heat, by increasing circulation. Don't overlook exercise, too, as a major factor in keeping the heart and small intestines in tune. Exercise will help make you sweat and eliminate some toxins from the blood, open up the old circulation and create new blood vessels (which provide increased blood flow to areas with restricted circulation).

Use the summertime to recharge yourself, balance the Water and Fire elements inside and out, and get plenty of physical activity and sunshine.

Summer Menus

1   Coconut Fish *Teriyaki* and Whole Vegetables on the Grill or Summer Kebabs
    Mixed Pepper Salad

2   *Aduki* Bean Rolls
    Five Heaps Noodles

3   Tofu Loaf
    Lemon Zucchini and Olives

4   Moroccan Vegetable Salad
    Stuffed Golden Nuggets

5   Gingered Noodled Soup
    Creamy Chicken Lasagne
    Bitter Green Salad

NOTE: The menus in this book serve 4-6 people.

Summer Menu 1: Coconut Fish *Teriyaki* and Whole Vegetables on the Barbeque or Summer Kebabs Mixed Pepper Salad

COCONUT FISH TERIYAKI

1 kg FISH FILLETS
LIME WEDGES AND FLAT-LEAF PARSLEY FOR GARNISH
Marinade
1 LARGE LIME
RICE OR BARLEY *MISO* OR SEA SALT TO TASTE
1 CUP MINCED SPRING ONIONS
2 t FINELY CHOPPED GINGER ROOT
1 GARLIC CLOVE CRUSHED (see snow pea arame salad, p 30)
1 SEEDED, MINCED GREEN CHILI PEPPER
1 SMALL BUNCH FRESH CORIANDER OR PARSLEY
1 t GROUND CUMIN
2 t GROUND CORIANDER
5 T DESICCATED OR 6 T GRATED FRESH COCONUT
1 T MAPLE SYRUP

1   Remove lime flesh, discarding seeds. Place lime flesh in blender or food processor and blend with miso, spring onions, ginger root, garlic, chili and fresh coriander or parsley until mixture is a smooth purée.

2   Add ground cumin and coriander, coconut and maple syrup and blend until mixture is smooth and creamy. Add a few drops of liquid if mixture is too thick, but do not make it too thin.

3   Put Marinade in a large dish and immerse the fish fillets, skin side up, for about 20 minutes.

4   Prepare barbeque.

5   When charcoal is medium hot, remove fish from Marinade and place on barbeque, skin side up. It is best to use an oiled wire fish basket,* which makes turning easier. Cook fillets for 5 minutes on each side or until the flesh flakes.

6   While fish cooks, strain Marinade into a small saucepan and reduce over medium heat by 1/3.

7   To serve, spoon some Marinade onto each plate and place fish on top. Garnish with flat leaf parsley and lime wedges.

* Available in Japanese shops.

S   U   M   M   E   R

WHOLE VEGETABLES ON THE BARBEQUE

CORN COBS

SUMMER SQUASH

POTATOES

Dressings

HERB-MARINATED OIL

OIL, VINEGAR AND FRESH HERB MARINADE (3 PARTS OIL: 1 PART VINEGAR)

Corn Cobs

With husks:

1 Soak corn ears in cold water for 30 – 90 minutes.

2 Place ears directly on charcoal, at edges of the barbeque. Cook for at least 30 minutes, turning often and sprinkling with cold water.

With husks and herb-marinated oil:

1 Soak corn ears in cold water for 30 – 90 minutes.

2 Peel husks back very carefully and baste ears with herb-marinated oil.

3 Replace husks and cook as above, but for at least 40 minutes. Prick the husks frequently with a fork while barbequing.

Without husks:

1 Wrap corn cobs in banana or lotus leaves (or foil if unavailable) and cook directly on charcoal for at least 30 minutes.

Summer Squash

1 If squash are long, cut in half lengthwise. If round, cut in half horizontally.

2 Brush skins with fresh herb marinade and cook directly on the barbeque for 15 – 20 minutes.

Potatoes

1 Wash potatoes well but do not peel. Prick all over with a fork and rub skins with oil.

2 Wrap in corn husks, banana leaves or lotus leaves (both available in Chinese stores), soaked in warm water for at least 1 hour beforehand.

3 Cook directly on the barbeque for at least 30 minutes.

SUMMER KEBABS

CHOICE OF VEGETABLES, FISH, SEAFOOD, CHICKEN, TOFU (OR TEMPEH), PLAIN OR MARINATED

Vegetable suggestions

ZUCCHINI CHUNKS

SQUASH CHUNKS

FRESH MUSHROOMS

SHALLOT BULBS

RED, YELLOW OR GREEN CAPSICUM QUARTERS, CUT INTO THIRDS
CROSSWAYS

LEBANESE CUCUMBER CHUNKS

BABY ONIONS (LIGHTLY PARBOILED)

PUMPKIN CHUNKS (LIGHTLY PARBOILED), 5 cm x 5 cm

CORN-ON-THE-COB CHUNKS (LIGHTLY PARBOILED), CUT IN QUARTERS
HORIZONTALLY

Marinade for Vegetables and Tofu

⅓ CUP OLIVE OIL

4 T *SHOYU* OR *TAMARI*

1 T MINCED GARLIC

1 T MINCED GINGER ROOT

4 T MINCED FRESH MARJORAM, OREGANO, BASIL OR THYME, OR 1 – 2 t DRIED

3 T CHOPPED CORIANDER OR PARSLEY LEAVES

Marinade for Fish, Seafood and Chicken

JUICE OF 1 LIME OR ½ ORANGE

1   Blend Marinade ingredients thoroughly.

2   Marinate fish and seafood for up to 6 hours.

3   Marinate chicken and vegetables for up to 12 hours.

4   Marinate tofu or tempeh for up to 24 hours.

5   If using bamboo skewers, soak for 30 minutes before threading kebabs.

7   Prepare barbeque.

8   Thread skewers with desired combinations.

9   Brush barbeque with a little oil and cook kebabs for 10 – 15 minutes or until tender. Turn and baste with marinade while cooking.

* Grilling may be used instead of barbeque method.

MIXED PEPPER SALAD

4 CAPSICUM PEPPERS OF DIFFERENT COLOURS

LEBANESE CUCUMBERS THINLY SLICED FOR GARNISH

Dressing

3 T OLIVE OIL

2 t BROWN RICE VINEGAR

2 GARLIC CLOVES CRUSHED (see snow pea arame salad, p 30)

SEA SALT AND FRESHLY GROUND PEPPER TO TASTE

S	U	M	M	E	R

1   Roast and peel capsicums (see split pea soup, p. 31). Cut into 2.5 cm strips.

2   Blend Dressing ingredients until well emulsified.

3   Spoon over capsicum strips and let sit for at least 60 minutes.

4   To serve, arrange cucumber slices on plates and decorate with the capsicum strips.

Summer Menu 2:   Aduki Bean Rolls
Five Heaps Noodles

ADUKI BEAN ROLLS

2 CUPS DRY *ADUKI* BEANS, SOAKED OVERNIGHT IN WATER TO COVER BY AT LEAST 5 cm

2 GARLIC CLOVES CRUSHED, MARINATED IN 2 T OIL

1 CUP DICED ONIONS

½ – ¾ CUP TAHINI OR ALMOND BUTTER

1 t GROUND CUMIN

2 – 3 T LEMON JUICE

½ CUP CHOPPED PARSLEY

ROASTED UNHULLED SESAME SEEDS FOR GARNISH

Forward planning: Aduki *beans may be cooked in advance.*

1   Drain Aduki beans and discard soaking water. Cover them with water by at least 3 cm and bring to the boil. Simmer for 20 minutes uncovered, skimming off residue that rises to the top.

2   Add more water if necessary. Cover the saucepan and cook the beans for about 1 more hour until they are soft. Alternatively, pressure cook them for about ½ hour.

3   Drain the beans and mash them well.

4   Heat dry wok or skillet and sauté the oil and garlic mixture briefly. Remove garlic. Add onions, cover and simmer until soft.

5   Blend ⅓ cup mashed beans with the onion and garlic mixture. Combine with the remaining beans, tahini or almond butter, cumin, lemon juice and parsley until smooth and well blended.

6   When the mixture is cool, shape into two logs and roll in sesame seeds. Slice and serve.

FIVE HEAPS NOODLES

150 g BROWN RICE NOODLES *BIFUN*

16 LARGE GRATED RADISHES

2 CUPS GRATED PUMPKIN

1 HEAD CHOPPED CURLY ENDIVE

OIL AS NEEDED

2 CUPS FRESH MUNG BEAN SPROUTS

¼ CUP *ARAME*

2 T TOASTED BLACK SESAME SEEDS FOR GARNISH (OPTIONAL)

Dressing

2 T TAHINI, ALMOND OR HAZELNUT PASTE

2 T JUICE OR WATER

1 T *SHOYU* OR *TAMARI*

2 – 3 t BROWN RICE VINEGAR

½ t JAPANESE LEMON PEPPER OR FRESHLY GROUND BLACK PEPPER

SEA SALT TO TASTE

2 T OIL

Forward planning: *Dressing should be made at least one day in advance.*

Dressing

1   Blend paste, juice or water, shoyu *or* tamari, *vinegar, pepper and sea salt together.*

2   Add oil in a thin stream and blend until the mixture is well emulsified.

Noodles

3   Pour boiling water over noodles to cover and set aside for 30 minutes.

4   Drain noodles and rinse under cold running water until cold. Chop into 5 cm lengths.

Five Heaps

5   Prepare radishes and pumpkin and curly endive.

6   Toss grated radishes and pumpkin in oil, keeping separate.

7   Drop bean sprouts into boiling unsalted water for 1 minute. Drain immediately and rinse under cold running water. Dry.

8   Wash arame *well and soak in water to cover for 3 minutes. Boil in soaking water for 5 minutes. Drain and dry.*

To serve:

9   Toss noodles gently with the Dressing.

10   Mould noodles in centre of large platter and surround with Five Heaps.

11   Garnish with sesame seeds.

S U M M E R

Summer Menu 3: Tofu Loaf
Lemon Zucchini and Olives

TOFU LOAF

700 g TOFU, DRAINED AND CRUMBLED
1½ CUPS COOKED BROWN RICE OR OTHER COOKED GRAIN
⅔ CUP FINELY CHOPPED PINE NUTS OR BLANCHED ALMONDS
⅔ CUP FINELY CHOPPED LIGHTLY TOASTED SUNFLOWER SEEDS
⅔ CUP FINELY CHOPPED LIGHTLY TOASTED HAZELNUTS
½ CUP OIL, TAHINI OR NUT BUTTER
½ CUP *MISO*, OR ¼ CUP *SHOYU* OR *TAMARI*, OR SEA SALT TO TASTE
½ CUP WHEATGERM OR NUTRITIONAL YEAST
4 T CHOPPED PARSLEY OR CORIANDER LEAVES
2 t LIGHTLY TOASTED CUMIN SEEDS, CRUSHED LIGHTLY
Sauce
2 T OIL
2 T WHOLEWHEAT, BARLEY OR BROWN RICE FLOUR
1 CUP SOYMILK OR ALMOND MILK (SEE BELOW)
3 T WHITE *MISO*, OR 4 T *SHOYU, TAMARI* AND SEA SALT TO TASTE
3 T TAHINI OR NUT BUTTER
½ CUP GRATED CARROT
1 CUP FINELY CHOPPED SHALLOTS OR CORIANDER LEAVES FOR GARNISH
Almond Milk (*alternative to soymilk for sauce above*)
½ CUP GROUND BLANCHED ALMONDS
1 CUP WATER
1 t MAPLE SYRUP

Forward planning: *Preheat oven to 180℃. Cook brown rice or other grain. Make almond milk.*

Almond Milk

1   Blend water and maple syrup into ground almonds until milk is desired consistency. Strain through washed muslin.

Tofu Loaf

2   Combine all ingredients and blend well. Do not overmix or it will be too creamy.

3   Spoon the mixture into an oiled loaf pan. Bake for 30 minutes or until the Loaf is set.

4   Alternatively, spoon the mixture into oiled individual moulds, cover each mould and steam in covered pan for 20 minutes or until set.

Sauce

5 Heat skillet, add oil and flour and cook over low heat several minutes, stirring continuously to avoid burning the mixture.

6 Heat soymilk or Almond Milk and add to mixture gradually, stirring continuously.

7 Add miso (creamed in a little water), and cook Sauce until thickened.

8 Blend in tahini or nut butter and grated carrot.

To serve:

9 Unmould tofu loaf or individual moulds and spoon Sauce over. Garnish with finely chopped shallots or coriander leaves.

LEMON ZUCCHINI and OLIVES

12 BRINE-CURED BLACK OLIVES, RINSED AND DRIED, OR OTHER PICKLES

6 SMALL ZUCCHINI

6 SMALL YELLOW SQUASH

3 T OIL

SEA SALT

1 T FINELY GRATED LEMON RIND

1 Pit olives and cut into quarters lengthwise.

2 Cut zucchini into quarters lengthwise, remove seeds if necessary, and slice into 6 mm pieces on the diagonal.

3 Cut squash into quarters and slice into 6 mm pieces on the diagonal.

4 Heat skillet, add oil and sauté zucchini and squash until tender, stirring frequently. Season with sea salt to taste.

5 Stir in olive quarters and heat through.

6 Remove from heat, add grated lemon rind and toss well. Adjust seasoning to taste.

S U M M E R

Summer Menu 4: Moroccan Vegetable Salad
Stuffed Golden Nuggets

MOROCCAN VEGETABLE SALAD

2 CUPS COUSCOUS

½ CUP CURRANTS OR CHOPPED SULTANAS

2 CUPS STOCK

½ CUP OLIVE OIL

½ CUP PINE NUTS

1 t TOASTED GROUND CUMIN SEEDS

1 t TOASTED GROUND CORIANDER SEEDS

3 CUPS THINLY SLICED SPRING ONIONS OR SHALLOTS

2 CUPS CHOPPED ZUCCHINI OR SUMMER SQUASH

2 SKINNED, FINELY CHOPPED YELLOW OR RED CAPSICUMS (see split pea soup, p. 31)

SEA SALT

4 – 5 T LEMON OR LIME JUICE

BLANCHED PEACH SLICES AND FRESH MINT LEAVES FOR GARNISH

1 Combine couscous and dried fruit in a bowl. Bring stock to the boil and pour over the mixture. Cover and leave for 5 minutes or until the stock is fully absorbed.

2 Heat skillet, add oil and sauté pine nuts until lightly browned. Remove with slotted spoon and set aside.

3 Add spices and shallots or spring onions to the oil and sauté until transparent.

4 Add zucchini or squash and sauté for a few minutes.

5 Add capsicums and sauté for a few minutes.

6 Lightly toss couscous mixture to fluff up the grains and add it to the pan for a few more minutes. Season with sea salt to taste.

7 Remove from heat and add lemon or lime juice and pine nuts.

8 Serve cold or at room temperature. Toss mixture lightly and garnish with mint leaves and peach slices.

STUFFED GOLDEN NUGGETS

2 GOLDEN NUGGET SQUASH

2 T GROUND *KUZU* OR ARROWROOT

350 g TOFU

3 T FINELY MINCED DILL PICKLES OR OTHER PICKLES

3 T FINELY MINCED CHINESE BLACK MUSHROOMS, SOAKED 4 HOURS AND

STALKS DISCARDED
2 T FINELY MINCED CARROTS
½ T FINELY MINCED SHALLOTS
2 t ROASTED SESAME OIL
½ T GROUND *KUZU* OR ARROWROOT
1 EGG WHITE
6 T OIL
SEA SALT
BROWN RICE MALT SYRUP (OPTIONAL)
¾ CUP STOCK

1   Cut golden nuggets lengthwise and scoop out all but 1 cm thickness of the flesh. The scooped-out flesh may be kept for later use. Blanch 4 – 5 minutes in boiling water or until half-cooked.

2   Coat the insides of the golden nugget halves with ½ T kuzu or arrowroot.

3   Blanch tofu by dropping into boiling water and draining well.

4   Break tofu into chunks and blend with pickles, mushrooms, carrots, shallots, sesame oil, kuzu or arrowroot and egg white.

5   Stuff golden nuggets with the mixture.

6   Heat skillet, add oil and add golden nuggets (stuffing-side down) for 2 minutes.

7   Add sea salt and brown rice malt syrup to taste. Cook for another minute.

8   Pour in the stock, cover pan and simmer golden nuggets for a further 7 – 8 minutes or until soft.

9   Serve on mignonette lettuce leaves.

S U M M E R

Summer Menu 5: Gingered Noodle Soup
Creamy Chicken Lasagne
Bitter Green Salad

GINGERED NOODLE SOUP

100 g MUNG BEAN CELLOPHANE NOODLES OR 1 GENEROUS CUP THIN WHOLEMEAL SPAGHETTI, BROKEN INTO 7 cm LENGTHS

2 T OIL

2 GARLIC CLOVES MINCED

2 t MINCED PEELED GINGER ROOT

1 CUP VERY THINLY SLICED ONION

1 CUP CARROT FLOWERS OR OTHER SHAPES, 2.5 cm IN DIAMETER

1 THINLY SLICED RED, YELLOW OR GREEN CAPSICUM

3 CUPS STOCK

1½ CUPS WATER

1 T *SHOYU* OR *TAMARI*

1 CUP THINLY SLICED CHICKEN MEAT (OPTIONAL)

1 CUP SHREDDED WATERCRESS LEAVES

½ CUP THINLY SLICED MUSHROOMS

1 CUP STRINGED SNOW PEAS

ROASTED SESAME OIL

BROWN RICE VINEGAR

SEA SALT AND JAPANESE CHILI PEPPER

1 CUP THINLY SLICED SHALLOTS FOR GARNISH

1   If using noodles, cover with boiling water and stand for 5 minutes. If using spaghetti, cook in boiling water until al dente — tender but firm. For both, rinse under cold running water, drain and set aside.

2   Heat wok or saucepan, add oil and stir fry garlic and ginger briefly. Add onions and cook until transparent. Add carrots, capsicum, stock, water and shoyu or tamari. Bring to the boil, cover and boil for 2 minutes.

3   Add optional chicken, watercress, mushrooms and noodles. Bring back to the boil, cover, turn off heat and let stand for 2 minutes.

4   Add snow peas and let stand a further couple of minutes until peas are crisp-tender.

5   Stir in roasted oil, vinegar, sea salt and chili pepper to taste.

6   To serve, ladle into bowls and garnish with shallots.

MACROBIOTICS & BEYOND

CREAMY CHICKEN LASAGNE

250 – 350 g. WHOLEWHEAT LASAGNE

NORI SHEETS

Chicken Sauce

2 CUPS UNCOOKED CHICKEN MINCE

3 T OIL AND 1 CUP OIL

SEA SALT AND FRESHLY GROUND BLACK PEPPER

5 – 6 CUPS STOCK

1 CUP BROWN RICE FLOUR

1½ CUPS FIRMLY PACKED BASIL LEAVES

1 CUP PINE NUTS

WHITE *MISO*

JAPANESE CHILI PEPPER

Mushrooms

500 g BUTTON MUSHROOMS

1 CUP FINELY CHOPPED ONIONS

1 t FINELY CHOPPED GARLIC

4 T CHOPPED PARSLEY

¼ t CHOPPED TARRAGON

½ CUP *MIRIN*

2 T OIL

SEA SALT OR *MISO*

Forward planning: *Preheat oven to 190°C. Mushrooms may be prepared in advance and kept covered in refrigerator.*

Chicken Sauce

1   Heat wok or skillet, add 3 T oil and sauté chicken mince until just opaque. Season with sea salt and pepper and set aside.

2   Bring stock to the boil in a saucepan.

3   Heat wok or skillet, add ½ cup oil and sauté brown rice flour over low heat for 4 – 5 minutes, stirring continuously.

4   Remove flour from heat and quickly add 5 cups of stock, stirring the mixture continuously until thick and creamy. Add more stock if the mixture is too thick, or boiling water if stock is finished. Cover and simmer 10 – 15 minutes, making sure the sauce does not burn.

5   Chop basil leaves finely in blender and blend in pine nuts. Add ½ cup oil in a thin stream, blending until the mixture is smooth and creamy. Add miso to taste.

6   Beat the basil and pine nut mixture into the hot sauce. Add the chicken. Season with sea salt and Japanese chili pepper.

SUMMER

Mushrooms
7 Wash mushrooms and trim stems.
8 Combine all the other ingredients in a saucepan and add mushrooms. Bring to the boil, cover and simmer for 8 – 10 minutes or until mushrooms are soft.

Pasta
9 Cook required number of lasagne sheets in boiling salted water until al dente — tender but firm. Rinse under cold running water and drain.

To combine
10 Fill lasagne dish with alternating layers of nori, Chicken Sauce, pasta and mushrooms. Cover the final layer of mushrooms with Chicken Sauce.
11 Cook in 190°C oven for 15 – 20 minutes.
12 Serve at room temperature.

BITTER GREEN SALAD

7 CUPS LETTUCE, RADICCHIO, CURLY ENDIVE AND CHICORY
6 T CHOPPED LIGHTLY TOASTED WALNUTS
Dressing
¼ CUP BROWN RICE VINEGAR
SEA SALT AND FRESHLY GOUND BLACK PEPPER
2 t COARSE GRAIN PREPARED MUSTARD
¾ CUP OIL
1 T CHOPPED FRESH OREGANO OR 1 t DRIED OREGANO

1 Whisk vinegar with sea salt, pepper and mustard. Add oil in a thin stream, blending until mixture is well emulsified. Add oregano and blend a few seconds longer.
2 Combine greens and walnuts in salad bowl and toss with the Dressing.

LATE SUMMER

Transitions are a part of life and every year we make adjustments when we change from one season to another. Late summer, associated with the Earth element in Chinese five-element theory, is the time of the year when we shift from outward to inward expression. Earth is the ground on which we stand and lay to rest, and it provides us with the food that nourishes and nurtures our well-being. It is central to all the other elements and in the Chinese system it is also called 'doyo', meaning 'transition'.

Late summer is a time when there is a tendency to change our food intake by increasing our protein foods and cooked foods, and perhaps including more dried foods, depending upon where we live and the work that we are presently engaged in. The organs relating to this time of the year are the stomach and spleen, which work hand-in-hand to digest food and distribute the energy from this food throughout our bodies.

There are four major transitionary times of the year which take place in between the seasons: when we change from winter to spring, spring to summer, summer to autumn and autumn to winter. There is usually a two or three-week transitionary time, around the two solstices and two equinoxes; when the weather can be very changeable and extreme in nature and temperature. During these transitional periods, it is vital that we remain centred and 'grounded' (maintaining contact with the Earth), so that inwardly we remain quiet and calm. Centring can also mean finding your own particular balance between Yin and Yang, Heaven and Earth, inner and outer, up and down, left and right.

Exercise is a positive way to maintain that balance, regulate your weight and maintain strength and vitality. Diet is also relevant, and as late summer is the beginning of harvest time, beans, apples, tomatoes, grapes and zucchini are just a few examples of Nature's abundance and gifts at this time of the year.

This is the time of the year for a 'building' diet, which includes a little more fat and protein than during the spring and summertime, and more warming and cooked foods. Increasing fish and poultry, if you are so inclined, will add to the potency of the 'building' diet. Continue it into the autumn and wintertime if you wish, so that you can feel stronger and warmer. During the seasonal transitions it is also advisable to take a few days to cleanse with juices, total fasting or just cutting down all intake by 50 per cent.

You will probably note some positive changes and easier 'transitions' as you become aware of your diet and exercise routine during the whole of the year. The way we feel daily, the way we cope with our work and family, how we sleep and relate

L   A   T   E   S   U   M   M   E   R

to the rest of the world emotionally, physically and spiritually are all dependent on centring ourselves in relation to the elements around us.

Late Summer Menus

1   Coconut Prawns with Peach Relish
    Millet and Split Pea Loaf

2   Chickpea Macadamia Soup
    Corn and Rice Combo

3   Butternut Spice
    Fish Exotica
    Sesame Spinach

4   Vegetable Tofu Quiche
    Spinach Crowns and Ginger Stir Fry

5   Bulghur Timbales
    Vegetable Kebabs
    Fig and Endive Salad

NOTE: The menus in this book serve 4 – 6 people.

Late Summer Menu 1:   Coconut Prawns with Peach Relish
Millet and Split Pea Loaf

COCONUT PRAWNS

20 – 24 FRESH UNCOOKED PRAWNS
SHREDDED COCONUT AS NEEDED
OIL FOR DEEP-FRYING
Batter
1½ CUPS CHICKPEA FLOUR (BESAN)
1 CUP WARM LIGHT BEER
2 T OIL
2 t CRUSHED GARLIC (see snow pea arame salad, p 30)
2 t GROUND CUMIN
½ t TURMERIC
SEA SALT AND FRESHLY GROUND BLACK PEPPER TO TASTE

63

MACROBIOTICS & BEYOND

1 Combine Batter ingredients and beat until smooth and free of lumps. Cover and set aside for 30 minutes.

2 Shell prawns, leaving tails intact.

3 Heat oil in wok or pan to deep frying temperature (180° – 190°C). (See p. 128 for deep-frying method.)

4 Holding by the tail, dip each prawn into batter; let excess batter drip off, and roll in shredded coconut.

5 Deep fry prawns for 2 – 3 minutes, taking care not to overcrowd pan. Drain well on rack or absorbent paper.

6 Keep prawns warm in a low over until ready to serve. Serve with Peach Relish.

PEACH RELISH

600 g FRESH PEACHES
½ CUP FRESH SPEARMINT LEAVES
¾ CUP BASIL LEAVES
2 T GROUND CORIANDER
2 t GROUND CUMIN
1 t GROUND GINGER OR 1 T GINGER JUICE (see p. 127)
½ – ¾ t JAPANESE SEVEN-SPICE CHILI POWDER
2 T MAPLE SYRUP OR TO TASTE
SEA SALT TO TASTE

Forward planning: May be made in advance, but do not add chili until serving. Relish will keep in refrigerator in sterilised glass jars for up to three weeks.

1 Blanch and peel peaches and chop into bite-sized pieces.

2 Blend all ingredients together to a smooth purée. Adjust seasoning.

3 Serve chilled with Coconut Prawns.

MILLET AND SPLIT PEA LOAF

⅔ CUP YELLOW SPLIT PEAS, SOAKED OVERNIGHT IN WATER TO COVER BY AT LEAST 5 cm
5 T OIL
1 t MUSTARD SEEDS
2 GARLIC CLOVES FINELY CHOPPED
2 CUPS THINLY SLICED ONION
2 CUPS HULLED MILLET
2 t GROUND CORIANDER

L A T E S U M M E R

1 t GROUND CUMIN

1 t TURMERIC OR ½ t SAFFRON THREADS SOAKED IN 1 T WATER

SEA SALT AND FRESHLY GROUND BLACK PEPPER

3 CUPS STOCK OR WATER

Forward planning: *Soak peas overnight.*

1   Drain split peas and discard soaking water.

2   Heat skillet, add oil and sauté mustard seeds for a few seconds. Add garlic and onions and sauté until the onions are transparent.

3   Add split peas, millet, coriander, cumin, turmeric or saffron and sea salt and pepper to taste. Sauté all ingredients for a few minutes.

4   Add 3 cups stock or water to the pan and bring to the boil. Cover and simmer 30 – 40 minutes or until the peas are soft.

5   Remove cover and sprinkle a few T of stock or water over the mixture. Cover and cook another 5 minutes.

6   Rinse mould in cold water, mix millet and pea mixture thoroughly and spoon into mould. Set aside for at least 1 hour or until the mixture sets.

7   Unmould and serve loaf with pickles, sauce or yoghurt.

Late Summer Menu 2:   Chickpea Macadamia Soup
Corn and Rice Combo

CHICKPEA MACADAMIA SOUP

2 T OIL

1 CUP CHOPPED ONIONS

1 GARLIC CLOVE MINCED

½ CUPS WHOLE MACADAMIA NUTS

3 – 4 CUPS COOKED CHICKPEAS (see spiced chickpeas with mocchi topping, page 29, for cooking method; use 1 – 1½ cup dried chickpeas)

1 CUP STOCK

1 CUP SOYMILK

2 T MINCED FRESH DILL

SEA SALT AND FRESHLY GROUND BLACK PEPPER

FRESH HERBS OR SPROUTS FOR GARNISH

Forward planning: *Cook chickpeas.*

1   Heat skillet, add oil and sauté onions until transparent. Add garlic and nuts and sauté until onions are golden brown.

2   Transfer to saucepan with chickpeas, stock and soymilk, dill and sea salt and pepper to taste. Cover and simmer the soup for 30 minutes, adding more liquid if the consistency is too thick.

3   Blend half the soup until smooth and creamy. Return to the saucepan and adjust seasoning to taste.

4   To serve, garnish with herbs or sprouts.

CORN AND RICE COMBO

½ CUP DRIED BLACK CHINESE MUSHROOMS, SOAKED IN WATER TO COVER FOR 4 HOURS
¼ CUP *SHOYU* OR *TAMARI*
¼ CUP *MIRIN*
4 CUPS STOCK
2 CUPS TOASTED BROWN RICE
1 CUP CORN KERNELS
1 BAY LEAF
TOASTED SEEDS
MINCED GREENS

Forward planning: *Soak mushrooms. Toast rice in 180°C oven on a low-sided baking tray until lightly browned.*

1   Drain mushrooms and reserve soaking water. Slice caps thinly. Discard stems.

2   Combine shoyu or tamari and mirin in a small saucepan, add mushrooms and bring to the boil. Reduce liquid until none remains. Set mushrooms aside.

3   Bring stock to the boil in a saucepan, add rice, corn kernels and bay leaf. Cover and simmer for 40 minutes or until rice is cooked.

4   To serve, toss with mushrooms, toasted seeds and greens.

LATE SUMMER

Late Summer Menu 3: Butternut Spice
                            Fish Exotica
                            Sesame Spinach

BUTTERNUT SPICE

2 T OIL
1 T FINELY CHOPPED, PEELED GINGER ROOT
2 CUPS CHOPPED ONION
2 – 3 t GROUND CORIANDER
2 t GROUND CUMIN
1 t GROUND CINNAMON
4 CARDAMON SEEDS
2 WHOLE CLOVES
1 t CHILI PEPPER (OPTIONAL)
4 CUPS CHOPPED BUTTERNUT PUMPKIN
STOCK OR WATER
SEA SALT TO TASTE OR 1 T *MISO*
CORIANDER LEAVES AND RED CAPSICUM STRIPS FOR GARNISH

1   Heat dry wok or skillet, add oil and sauté finely chopped ginger root for a few seconds.
2   Add chopped onion and sauté until lightly browned.
3   Add spices one at a time and coat mixture well with oil.
4   Add chopped butternut pumpkin and coat mixture well with oil.
5   Add enought stock or water to barely cover the vegetables. Season to taste. If using miso, place the miso on top, but do not mix into the vegetables. Bring liquid to the boil, cover and simmer for 15 minutes or until the butternut is soft.
6   Garnish with coriander leaves and red capsicum strips.

FISH EXOTICA

500 g FIRM FLESHED, SKINNED FISH FILLETS
2 SLICES GINGER ROOT, CRUSHED WITH THE FLAT BLADE OF A KNIFE
1 T RICE WINE
SEA SALT TO TASTE
Sauce
2 T OIL

67

MACROBIOTICS & BEYOND

1 T MINCED FERMENTED BLACK BEANS, RINSED WHILE WHOLE OR MINCED OLIVES
1 T MINCED SHALLOTS
1 T MINCED GARLIC
¼ CUP FISH OR CHICKEN STOCK
1 T SHOYU OR TAMARI
1 T RICE WINE
1 t MAPLE SYRUP
¼ t JAPANESE LEMON PEPPER OR FRESHLY GROUND BLACK PEPPER
250 g MINCED SEAFOOD, STEAMED WITH FISH, FOR GARNISH

Forward planning: *Prepare sauce.*

To prepare fish

1   Rinse the fillets quickly and pat dry. Place in a bowl with ginger root, rice wine and sea salt, and marinate for 15 minutes.

2   Discard ginger root and place fillets on a heatproof platter.

To make Sauce

3   Heat dry wok or skillet, add oil and sauté black beans or olives, shallots and garlic for a few seconds.

4   Add stock, shoyu or tamari, rice wine, maple syrup and pepper. Bring to the boil and simmer for 2 minutes, stirring constantly.

To cook fish

5   Pour the Sauce over the fillets.

6   Place the platter in steamer, sprinkle seafood on top, cover and steam over boiling water for 10 minutes or until the fish flakes.

7   Re-arrange garnish before serving.

SESAME SPINACH

1 BUNCH ENGLISH SPINACH
4 T UNHULLED TOASTED SESAME SEEDS
1 T BROWN RICE MALT SYRUP OR MALTOSE
2 – 3 t SHOYU OR TAMARI
2 – 3 T STOCK

1   Wash spinach in a sink or bowl of water to remove all sand from stalks. Discard any slimy leaves. Remove and drain spinach.

2   Bring salted water to boil in a saucepan. Hold spinach leaves and immerse stalks for about 30 seconds. Immerse leaves and blanch for about 60 more seconds.

3   Drain spinach and rinse under cold running water to stop further cooking. Roll

L A T E S U M M E R

spinach in a towel or bamboo mat and squeeze out excess water.

4   Remove crowns (roots) and cut the spinach into 5 cm lengths.

5   Crush warmed toasted sesame seeds in a suribachi or mortar.

6   Combine rice syrup or maltose, shoyu or tamari and stock by warming them in a small saucepan. Add the mixture to the sesame seeds.

7   Put the spinach into the suribachi or mortar and toss with the dressing.

Late Summer Menu 4:   Vegetable Tofu Quiche
Spinach Crowns and Ginger Stir Fry

VEGETABLE TOFU QUICHE

Pastry

2 CUPS WHOLEMEAL PASTRY FLOUR

½ t SEA SALT

⅔ CUP BOILING WATER

¼ CUP OIL

Filling

2 T OIL

2 t MINCED GARLIC

1 T MINCED GINGER ROOT

2 CUPS CHOPPED SHALLOTS OR SPRING ONIONS

1 CUP CHOPPED FENNEL

1 CUP CHOPPED BRUSSELS SPROUTS

½ CUP DICED CARROTS

600 g TOFU

1 EGG OR 1 – 2 T GROUND *KUZU* OR ARROWROOT DISSOLVED IN 4 T COLD
WATER

SEA SALT OR *MISO* TO TASTE

4 T FRESH HERBS OR 1 t DRIED HERBS

Baking equipment *A pie dish or flan that will hold 5 cups of filling*

Forward planning: *Vegetables may be cooked in advance. Preheat oven to 180°C.*

Pastry

1   *Combine flour and sea salt in a bowl. Beat boiling water vigorously into oil until creamy. Add to dry ingredients all at once. Knead the mixture until the dough forms a ball, adding a little more water or flour if necessary. Wrap the dough well so that it does not dry out and rest in the refrigerator for 15 minutes.*

MACROBIOTICS & BEYOND

2   Roll the pastry very thinly on a sheet of greaseproof paper and invert over the oiled pie dish or flan, positioning the pastry to line the dish or flan evenly. Partially bake on the middle shelf of a 180°C oven for 10 minutes.

Filling

3   Heat dry wok or skillet, add oil, and sauté garlic, ginger root and shallots until the shallots are transparent. Add the fennel, brussels sprouts and carrots, cover the wok and cook over low heat until the vegetables are almost soft. Watch that the vegetables do not stick to the wok, adding a little water or stock if necessary.

4   Drop tofu into boiling water for 1 minute and drain well. Blend with the egg or dissolved kuzu, salt or miso and herbs, to form a smooth cream.

5   Combine the vegetables and tofu cream.

To cook quiche

6   Fill the pastry crust with the mixture. Bake in a 180°C for 30 minutes or until the quiche has risen and almost set. If you have used a deep dish, the quiche may need as much as 50 minutes to cook.

NOTE: Experiment with different combinations of vegetables, and with different proportions of vegetables and tofu cream, to discover your favourite combinations.

SPINACH CROWNS AND GINGER STIR FRY

1 T OIL
6 THIN SLICES PEELED GINGER ROOT, CUT IN JULIENNE STRIPS
SPINACH CROWNS FROM 1 BUNCH ENGLISH SPINACH, SLICED LENGTHWISE ON THE DIAGONAL
SEA SALT OR *SHOYU* TO TASTE
LEMON JUICE TO TASTE

Forward planning: *Wash and dry spinach crowns well. Trim them.*

1   Heat dry wok or skillet, add oil and briefly sauté ginger strips. Add the spinach crowns and stir fry until they are just soft.

2   Season with sea salt or shoyu and lemon juice.

L A T E   S U M M E R

Late Summer Menu 5: Bulghur Timbales
Vegetable Kebabs
Fig and Endive Salad

BULGHUR TIMBALES

2 T OIL
4 T THINLY SLICED SHALLOTS
1 CUP MINCED MUSHROOMS
1 CUP COARSE GRAIN BULGHUR
1 CUP STOCK
1 T FINELY GRATED LIME RIND
4 – 5 T FRESHLY SNIPPED CHIVES
SEA SALT AND JAPANESE LEMON PEPPER
1 LIME OR LEMON DECORATIVELY CUT FOR GARNISH

1   *Heat wok or skillet, add oil and sauté shallots until transparent.*

2   *Add mushrooms and sauté 1 – 2 minutes.*

3   *Stir in bulghur, add stock and bring to boil. Cover and simmer for 10 minutes or until bulghur is cooked.*

4   *Fluff bulghur lightly. Add lime rind and chives, cover and let stand off the heat for 5 minutes.*

5   *Season with sea salt and lemon pepper.*

6   *Pack bulghur into ½ cup oiled moulds and leave for 5 – 10 minutes.*

7   *To serve, invert a mould onto each plate and garnish with lime or lemon slices and chives.*

VEGETABLE KEBABS

12 SHALLOT BULBS CUT IN 7 cm LENGTH
6 ROUND YELLOW SQUASH, 2.5 – 3 cm IN DIAMETER, BLANCHED UNTIL ALMOST SOFT AND HALVED LENGTHWISE
4 JAPANESE (SLENDER) EGGPLANTS, HALVED LENGTHWISE
1 RED, YELLOW OR GREEN CAPSICUM, SEEDED AND QUARTERED, OR 12 THICK ZUCCHINI SLICES, 2.5 cm IN DIAMETER

Marinade

¼ CUP BROWN RICE VINEGAR
1 t COARSE GRAIN PREPARED MUSTARD
2 – 4 T *NATTO* (OR OTHER) *MISO*

¾ CUP OIL

2 T MINCED FRESH HERBS

Forward planning: *Prepare marinade and marinate.*
1 Combine all vegetables in a bowl.
2 Blend vinegar, mustard and miso together and add oil in a thin stream, blending until mixture is well emulsified. Stir in herbs.
3 Spoon Marinade over vegetables and let stand for 15 minutes or longer.
4 Prepare grill.
5 Arrange vegetables on skewers. (Pre-soak bamboo skewers in water for 30 minutes.)
6 Grill kebabs until kebabs are well cooked, basting occasionally with Marinade.

FIG AND ENDIVE SALAD

12 STALKS CURLY ENDIVE

½ CUP ALFALFA SPROUTS

2 FRESH RIPE FIGS, HALVED

PARSLEY SPRIGS FOR GARNISH

Dressing

½ CUP TOASTED GROUND BLANCHED ALMONDS

1 CUP MINCED SHALLOTS

½ CUP MINCED FRESH CORIANDER LEAVES

1 t GROUND CUMIN (OR TO TASTE)

1 – 2 T LEMON JUICE

½ CUP OIL

WATER AS NEEDED

1 Blend nuts, shallots, coriander, cumin and lemon juice together. Add oil slowly in a thin stream, adding water if necessary, until the Dressing is well emulsified and of desired consistency.
2 Arrange endive stalks, sprouts and fig halves on a plate.
3 Spoon dressing over the salad and garnish with parsley sprigs.

AUTUMN

Autumn provides a time for us to shift naturally from directing our energy outside the home, to directing it more towards our families, friends, work and indoor projects.

Conservation is the key word, not only in our social activities but also when it comes to food: harvesting, preserving and conserving become more significant, so that we can store the excess and enjoy the benefits during the winter months still to come.

Those of us who already eat less meat turn more towards vegetables and grains than fruit — especially as the winter grows colder. Become aware of the complex effects of foods on your body. The quantity and ratio of foods solely depends upon you and how they react in your system.

For example meats, which are basically concentrated energy and not easily assimilable, will create more heat and density than fruits, grains and vegetables. Cheese and bread, which are both congestors, will not allow your intestines to flow smoothly. Eating too much or too many congesting foods keeps you from developing a more acute awareness of your needs.

Vegetables and fruits are body cleansers, but certain fruits like bananas have a congesting effect. Mushrooms act as a body builder, as do fish, meat, dairy products, nuts, beans, seeds and grains — but these foods can produce some congestion as well.

Whole grains are the key to good elimination, and a diet consisting mainly of body cleansers, some building foods, and a limited intake of congestors will keep you feeling vital and strong. You must choose your diet in relation to your genetic heritage, activity, climate and lifestyle.

Autumn weather brings forth an opportunity to harvest pumpkin, squash, beans, cabbage, turnips, onions, garlic, rice, barley, celery, watercress and spinach, to name just a few. Baked squash or pumpkin stuffed with a combination of brown rice, sliced almonds, fish and mushrooms is a perfect meal to embrace the first crisp days of autumn and welcome Nature's bounty. Don't forget ginger root, which also makes its debut in early autumn and is so helpful for extra body heat and clearing the lungs. Either simmer it with water and drink as a tea, or dip a towel into the tea and apply it to congested areas to promote circulation.

Eating and lifestyle habits are crucial to your sense of well-being, development and growth. This autumn, take the time to assume responsibility for yourself from the inside, so that diseases don't force you to change your life, and your body and mind remain clear, positive and in balance for the seasons to come.

Autumn Menus

1   Leek Croquettes
    Haricot Bean Hotpot

2   Watercress *Miso* Soup
    Peanut Pumpkin Fritters

3   Lima Bean and Rosemary Soup
    Chestnut Rice
    Oriental Salad

4   Chicken or Fish Balls with Basil Sauce and Noodles
    Endive Beet Salad with Orange Caraway Vinaigrette

5   Walnut Broccoli
    Olive Chestnut Patties

NOTE: The menus in this book serve 4 – 6 people.

Autumn Menu 1:   Leek Croquettes
Haricot Bean Hotpot

LEEK CROQUETTES

4 – 4½ CUPS FINELY CHOPPED LEEKS, WHITE PART ONLY
2 EGGS
SEA SALT TO TASTE
JAPANESE LEMON PEPPER OR FRESHLY GROUND BLACK PEPPER TO TASTE
¼ – ½ CUP WHOLEMEAL BREADCRUMBS
OIL AS NEEDED
CURLY ENDIVE FOR GARNISH
Chili Dip
½ CUP BOILING WATER OR STOCK
⅔ CUP *SHOYU* OR *TAMARI*
JAPANESE RED PEPPER TO TASTE

Forward planning: *The croquette mixture may be prepared in the morning for cooking later in the day. Chili Dip base may be made in advance.*

A U T U M N

1 Put the finely chopped leeks in a saucepan and barely cover with water. Simmer the leeks until they are soft. Drain them well, pressing all the water out through the sieve with a large spoon.

2 Beat the eggs. Mix the leeks with the eggs, sea salt and pepper. Gradually add the breadcrumbs, until the mixture holds together when dropped from a spoon.

3 When the mixture is cool, form it into small croquettes. If making the croquettes in advance, cover the batter and form croquettes just before cooking.

4 Heat a skillet, add several T of oil as needed and cook the croquettes over medium heat until they are lightly browned on all sides.

5 To make Chili Dip: combine boiling water or stock with shoyu or tamari. Just before serving, sprinkle in chili to taste.

6 To serve croquettes, garnish with sprigs of curly endive and serve with Chili Dip.

HARICOT BEAN HOTPOT

1½ CUPS HARICOT BEANS, SOAKED OVERNIGHT IN WATER TO COVER BY AT LEAST 5 cm

12 PEELED AND CRUSHED GARLIC CLOVES (see snow arame salad, p. 30)

¼ CUP OIL

1 BAY LEAF

3 T CHOPPED FRESH OREGANO OR 1 t DRIED OREGANO

2 T UMEBOSHI PASTE OR TOMATO PASTE OR SAUCE

SEA SALT

JAPANESE LEMON PEPPER OR FRESHLY GROUND BLACK PEPPER TO TASTE

JUICE OF 1 LEMON (2 – 3 T)

1 CUP MINCED SHALLOTS FOR GARNISH

½ CUP FINELY CHOPPED PARSLEY FOR GARNISH

Forward planning: Soak beans in advance.

1 Drain the beans. Add fresh water to the beans in a saucepan, to cover by at least 3 cm. Bring to the boil, lower the heat and simmer, uncovered, for 20 minutes, skimming off residue that rises to the top.

2 Add the garlic, oil, bay leaf and oregano to the saucepan; cover, and simmer the beans for 1 hour or until they are soft. Alternatively, pressure cook them for 30 minutes.

3 Stir in the umeboshi or tomato paste, and sea salt and pepper to taste. Cook the beans gently, uncovered, for another 15 minutes or until the cooking liquid has evaporated.

4 To serve, stir the lemon juice into the beans and garnish with the shallots and parsley.

MACROBIOTICS & BEYOND

Autumn Menu 2: Watercress *Miso* Soup
Peanut Pumpkin Fritters

WATERCRESS MISO SOUP

3 CUPS STOCK
2 CUPS FIRMLY PACKED WATERCRESS LEAVES
1 ½ CUPS MINCED SHALLOTS
1 T GROUND *KUZU* OR ARROWROOT
2 – 3 t LEMON JUICE
SWEET WHITE *MISO* (1 t PER PERSON)
FINELY GRATED LEMON RIND FOR GARNISH

1   Bring the stock to the boil in a saucepan. Add the watercress and shallots and simmer for 5 minutes.

2   Strain the cooking liquid through a fine sieve into a bowl.

3   Purée the watercress and shallot mixture with ½ cup of the cooking liquid.

4   Dissolve the kuzu or arrowroot in ½ cup cold water.

5   Put the cooking liquid and purée into the saucepan. Add the dissolved kuzu or arrowroot and bring to the boil, stirring continuously. Add the lemon juice and miso.

6   To serve, garnish with finely grated lemon rind.

PEANUT PUMPKIN FRITTERS

1 CUP BROWN RICE FLOUR
1 T GROUND NUTS
1 CUP CHOPPED NUTS OR SEEDS
1 T GROUND *KUZU* OR ARROWROOT
1 t GROUND CORIANDER
SEA SALT TO TASTE
½ CUP GRATED ONION
1 CUP PUMPKIN PURÉE
½ CUP PEANUT BUTTER
SOYMILK OR WATER
OIL FOR DEEP-FRYING
Fresh Coriander Sauce
2 T GROUND *KUZU* OR ARROWROOT
1½ CUPS STOCK OR WATER
1 T *SHOYU* OR *TAMARI*

A	U	T	U	M	N

SEA SALT TO TASTE

1 T TOASTED BLACK SESAME SEEDS

2 T MINCED FRESH CORIANDER LEAVES

LEMON JUICE TO TASTE

1   Combine the rice flour, ground nuts, chopped nuts or seeds, kuzu, or arrowroot, coriander and sea salt.

2   Combine the onion, pumpkin and peanut butter.

3   Mix all the ingredients together, adding soymilk or water to make a smooth, thick batter.

4   Heat oil in a wok or pan to deep frying temperature (180° – 190°C) – see p.128 for deep-frying method. Drop the fritter batter by tablespoons into the oil and deep-fry until the fritters are golden on both sides. Do not overcrowd the pan or the oil temperature will fall too low for successful frying. Drain the fritters well on a rack or absorbent paper.

5   To make the Fresh Coriander Sauce: dissolve the kuzu or arrowroot in a saucepan with the cold stock or water and bring to the boil, stirring continously. Season with shoyu and tamari and sea salt. Remove from heat. Just before serving fritters, add sesame seeds, coriander and lemon juice.

6   Drop the drained fritters, a few at a time, into the simmering sauce. Remove when heated through and serve.

Autumn Menu 3:   Lima Bean and Rosemary Soup
Chestnut Rice
Oriental Salad

LIMA BEAN AND ROSEMARY SOUP

1 CUP DRY LIMA BEANS, SOAKED OVERNIGHT IN WATER TO COVER BY AT LEAST 5 cm

3 – 5 CUPS STOCK

1 BAY LEAF OR 1 x 15 cm STRIP *KOMBU*

4 T OIL

1 SPRIG FRESH ROSEMARY

1 – 2 GARLIC CLOVES

2 – 3 T FRESH PASTA SAUCE OR PASTE

SEA SALT TO TASTE

JAPANESE LEMON PEPPER OR FRESHLY GROUND PEPPER TO TASTE

Forward planning: *Soak lima beans overnight.*

1   Drain lima beans and discard soaking water. Cover the beans with stock by at least 3 cm and bring to the boil. Simmer for 20 minutes uncovered, skimming off residue that rises to the top.

2   Add more stock if necessary. Add the bay leaf or kombu, *cover saucepan and cook the beans for about 1 more hour until they are soft. Alternatively, pressure cook them for about ½ hour.*

3   Heat a dry wok or skillet, add the oil and sauté the rosemary sprig and garlic. When the garlic begins to brown, remove the garlic and rosemary sprig.

4   Add the pasta sauce diluted in boiling water, watching that it does not spit. Cover the pan and simmer slowly for 10 minutes.

5   Add the sauce to the lima beans and enough stock to cover them. (On a cold night, blend half the soup to make it thicker.) Season with sea salt and pepper and simmer the soup for 10 minutes.

6   Serve with wholemeal croutons.

CHESTNUT RICE

1 CUP DRIED CHESTNUTS, SOAKED OVERNIGHT IN BOILING WATER TO COVER BY AT LEAST 5 cm

3½ CUPS WATER, INCLUDING CHESTNUT SOAKING WATER

2 CUPS BROWN RICE

½ t SEA SALT

Forward planning: *Soak chestnuts overnight. Rice may be washed beforehand.*

1   Drain the chestnuts and add enough water to the chestnut soaking water to make 3½ cups.

2   Combine the water with the chestnuts, rice and sea salt in a saucepan, cover, bring to the boil and simmer for 50 minutes or until the rice is cooked. Alternatively, pressure cook for 45 minutes.

ORIENTAL SALAD

6 – 8 DRIED CHINESE BLACK MUSHROOMS, SOAKED FOR 4 HOURS

¼ CUP TAMARI *OR* SHOYU

½ CUP *MIRIN* OR RICE WINE

500 g BROCCOLI

3 CUPS THINLY SLICED RADISHES

½ CUP SHALLOTS SLICED ON THE DIAGONAL

A U T U M N

Oriental Dressing

½ CUP TOFU
1 GARLIC CLOVE CRUSHED
3 – 4 t BROWN RICE VINEGAR
FRESHLY GROUND BLACK PEPPER TO TASTE
SEA SALT TO TASTE
2 – 3 t ROASTED SESAME OIL
⅓ CUP OIL

Forward planning: *Soak mushrooms in water to cover. Dressing should be made at least one day in advance. Broccoli may be blanched in advance.*

Dressing

1 Drop tofu into boiling water for 1 minute and drain well.

2 Break tofu into pieces and blend with garlic, vinegar, pepper and sea salt until the mixture is smooth and creamy.

3 Add the oils in a thin stream until the mixture is well emulsified.

Salad

4 Drain mushrooms and discard stalks. Slice caps into thin strips.

5 Bring tamari or shoyu and mirin or rice wine to the boil in a small saucepan. Add mushrooms strips and simmer until the liquid has evaporated. Cool.

6 Separate the broccoli head into bite-sized florets. Peel the stalks and slice thinly on the diagonal. Drop the stalk pieces into boiling salted water and blanch for 2 – 3 minutes. Remove. In a strainer, blanch the florets in the water until they turn bright green. Drain, rinse under cold running water and dry.

7 To serve, arrange mushrooms, broccoli, radishes and shallots on a rectangular plate, in alternating diagonal rows. Spoon the Dressing over the vegetables.

MACROBIOTICS & BEYOND

Autumn Menu 4: Chicken or Fish Balls with Basil Sauce and Noodles
Endive Beet Salad with Orange Caraway Vinaigrette

CHICKEN OR FISH BALLS WITH BASIL SAUCE AND NOODLES

350 g GROUND UNCOOKED CHICKEN OR FISH
2 – 3 T MINCED ONION
½ t GINGER JUICE
1 t *MISO*
SEA SALT TO TASTE
1 t GROUND *KUZU* OR ARROWROOT, OR AS NEEDED
OIL FOR DEEP-FRYING
250 g DRIED OR 500 g FRESH DELICATE WHOLEMEAL NOODLES
Basil Sauce
600 g TOFU
1 CUP GROUND PINE NUTS OR BLANCHED ALMONDS
½ CUP MINCED FRESH BASIL
½ CUP MINCED FRESH PARSLEY
SEA SALT TO TASTE
½ CUP OLIVE OIL OR ⅓ CUP SOYA MAYONNAISE

Forward planning: *Sauce should be made at least one day in advance. Noodles may be cooked in advance.*

Basil Sauce

1 Drop the tofu into boiling water for 1 minute and drain well. Break it into pieces and blend with the nuts, basil, parsley and sea salt until the mixture is smooth and creamy.

2 Add the oil slowly in a thin stream, or the mayonnaise gradually, and blend to a smooth sauce. Thin the sauce with a little stock or water if necessary when using.

Chicken or Fish Balls

3 Combine the chicken or fish, onion, ginger juice (made by grating fresh ginger root on a porcelain grater or the smallest holes of a steel grater), miso and sea salt thoroughly in a bowl until well blended. Sprinkle the kuzu or arrowroot over the mixture, leave for about 10 minutes, and then mix it.

4 Oil hands and shape the mixture into balls the size of a walnut in the shell.

5 Heat oil in a wok or pan to deep frying temperature (180° – 190°C) – See p.128 for deep-frying method. Drop the balls into the oil and deep fry for 3 – 4 minutes or

A   U   T   U   M   N

until they are golden all over. Do not overcrowd the pan or the oil temperature will fall too low for successful frying. Drain well on a rack or absorbent paper.

6   Bring a large saucepan of water the boil. Drop in the noodles gradually so that they do not stick together.

7   Bring noodles to the boil, stirring occasionally. As they come up to the boil, add just enough cold water to stop them boiling.

8   Repeat this action two more times.

9   Let noodles come to the boil and simmer them until they are cooked al dente — tender but firm. Drain. If cooking noodles in advance, drain and rinse under cold running water until cold, and reheat to serve.

To serve:

10   Place the chicken or fish balls on the noodles and spoon Basil Sauce over them.

ENDIVE BEET SALAD WITH ORANGE CARAWAY VINAIGRETTE

2 - 3 HEAD BELGIAN ENDIVE (WITLOOF), TRIMMED AND SEPARATED INTO SINGLE LEAVES

1 HEAD CURLY ENDIVE, TRIMMED OF COARSE STEMS

BEETROOT (TO MAKE 2 CUPS OF THIN SLICES WHEN COOKED)

Orange Caraway Vinaigrette

1 t LIGHTLY TOASTED CARAWAY SEEDS

2 t PREPARED MUSTARD

2 T LEMON JUICE OR BROWN RICE VINEGAR

1 T ORANGE JUICE

SEA SALT TO TASTE

JAPANESE LEMON PEPPER OR FRESHLY GROUND BLACK PEPPER TO TASTE

¾ CUP SESAME OIL

1 t FINELY GRATED ORANGE RIND

1 T MINCED FRESH CORIANDER LEAVES

3 T MINCED FRESH PARSLEY

½ CUP GRATED APPLE

Forward planning: *The Vinaigrette should be made at least one day in advance, to enhance flavour. Beetroot can be cooked in advance.*

1   Pressure cook whole beetroots for about 20 minutes, depending on size. Alternatively, bake them whole in a covered pan with a little water in a 190°C oven for at least 1 hour. Cool, peel and slice.

To make Vinaigrette

2   Grind the caraway seeds; blend them with the mustard, lemon juice or vinegar,

MACROBIOTICS & BEYOND

orange juice and sea salt and pepper until the mixture is creamy. Add the oil slowly in a thin stream and blend until the dressing is well emulsified. Add the orange rind, coriander, parsley and apple, and blend a few seconds more.

3   Arrange 5 Belgian endive leaves on each plate in a spoke pattern. Top them with shredded curly endive. Arrange beetroot slices over the curly endive. Spoon the Vinaigrette over the salad.

Autumn Menu 5:   Walnut Broccoli
Olive Chestnut Patties

WALNUT BROCCOLI

500 g BROCCOLI
Sauce
⅔ CUP GROUND WALNUTS
3 T *MIRIN* OR RICE WINE
3 T *SHOYU* OR *TAMARI*, OR 2 T MISO
WATER OR COOKING LIQUID AS NEEDED
JAPANESE 7 SPICE CHILI PEPPER TO TASTE

Forward planning: *Broccoli and Sauce may be prepared in advance and kept separate.*

1   Separate broccoli head into bite-sized florets. Peel stalks and slice thinly on the diagonal. Drop stalk pieces into boiling salted water and blanch for 2 – 3 minutes. Remove. In a strainer, blanch the florets in the boiling water until they turn bright green. Drain, rinse under cold running water and dry.

2   Combine the Sauce ingredients in a small saucepan, bring to the boil and simmer for 1 – 2 minutes until creamy. Set aside to cool.

3   To serve, toss the broccoli with the Sauce.

OLIVE PATTIES

2 CUPS COOKED CHESTNUT RICE (see p. 78) OR PLAIN COOKED RICE
½ CUP CHOPPED PITTED OLIVES
2 T GROUND NUTS OR SEEDS (IF NOT USING CHESTNUT RICE)
4 T MINCED FRESH PARSLEY
1 t MIXED DRIED HERBS

82

A U T U M N

SEA SALT TO TASTE
1 – 2 T OIL
LETTUCE OR RADICCHIO LEAVES FOR GARNISH

1 Combine Chestnut Rice or plain rice, olives, nuts or seeds (if used), parsley, mixed herbs, sea salt and 1 t oil. Using a blender or food processor if rice is very dry, bind the mixture. (Alternatively, if rice is dry, use cooked oatmeal to get the same result; or add a few drops of stock or water and bind with 1 – 2 t of ground kuzu or arrowroot.)
2 Shape the mixture into patties 5 cm in diameter and 60 mm thick.
3 Heat dry skillet, add remaining oil and fry the patties until lightly browned on both sides. Alternatively, grill them until lightly browned.
4 Serve on lettuce or radicchio leaves, with mustard or pickles.

COLD DESSERTS

Soy Custard
Cherry Carob Pudding
Strawberry Mousse
Fruit Freezes

SOY CUSTARD

2 CUPS SCALDED SOYMILK
1 T OIL
2 EGGS (AT ROOM TEMPERATURE)
¼ CUP MAPLE SYRUP
½ t VANILLA

1   *Heat soymilk and beat oil into it.*
2   *Beat eggs until frothy and gradually beat in maple syrup.*
3   *Still beating, add hot milk in a thin stream. Add vanilla.*
4   *Pour mixture into an oiled baking dish or individual moulds. Place in shallow pan of water and bake at 160°C for 35 – 40 minutes or until the custard is set.*

CHERRY CAROB PUDDING

500 g FRESH CHERRIES
4 T AGAR-AGAR FLAKES
2 CUPS APPLE JUICE
4 T TAHINI OR CASHEW NUT BUTTER
3 T GROUND *KUZU* OR ARROWROOT FLOUR
PINCH SEA SALT OR ½ T WHITE *MISO*
5 T ROASTED CAROB POWDER
5 T MAPLE SYRUP
3 T MALTOSE (OPTIONAL) OR BROWN RICE MALT SYRUP
2 t VANILLA OR FINELY GRATED ORANGE RIND
¼ CUP FINELY CHOPPED ALMONDS

1   *Pit cherries and set aside.*
2   *Combine agar-agar and apple juice in saucepan and bring to the boil. Lower heat and simmer until agar-agar dissolves.*

C O L D   D E S S E R T S

3 Cream tahini or cashew nut butter with kuzu or arrowroot and sea salt or miso. Blend into liquid.

4 Add carob, maple syrup and optional maltose or rice syrup, and simmer for 10 minutes.

5 Remove from heat and stir in cherries, vanilla or orange rind and almonds. Cool until set.

6 Serve as is, or blend one-half of the pudding to a cream, chop the remaining half into small cubes and fold them into the cream mixture.

STRAWBERRY MOUSSE

2 CUPS STRAWBERRIES (2 PUNNETS)

5 T AGAR-AGAR FLAKES

1½ CUPS APPLE JUICE OR 1 CUP APPLE JUICE AND ½ CUP *MIRIN*

½ CUP TOFU

1 T TAHINI

¼ CUP MAPLE SYRUP

1 EGG WHITE (AT ROOM TEMPERATURE)

1 Wash and hull strawberries and cut in halves.

2 Combine agar-agar and apple juice in saucepan and bring to the boil. Lower heat and simmer until agar-agar dissolves.

3 Combine strawberries and liquid with tofu and tahini and blend until smooth and creamy.

4 Heat maple syrup to 'soft ball' stage (116°C) — use candy thermometer or boil 5 - 8 minutes or until syrup looks like caramel.

5 Beat egg white with a pinch of salt to form stiff peaks. Still beating, drip in hot maple syrup. Fold egg white carefully into strawberry mixture.

6 Place into serving dishes and chill. Decorate with sliced strawberries.

FRUIT FREEZES

Berry and Banana Freeze

3 VERY RIPE BANANAS WITH BROWN SKIN

2 CUPS STRAWBERRIES OR BLUEBERRIES (2 PUNNETS)

1 Blend fruit together to a purée and freeze. Remove every half hour or so, 2 or 3 times, and blend or stir before freezing again.

2 Alternatively, freeze in ice-cream machine or blend fruit together and refrigerate until chilled (the thick rich consistency of the puree allowing it to set without freezing).

Blackberry and Apricot or Peach Freeze

2 CUPS BLACKBERRIES
5 PEACHES or 12 – 15 APRICOTS, PITTED
MAPLE SYRUP TO TASTE

Prepare as above.

Passionfruit Surprise

10 VERY RIPE PASSIONFRUIT
1 VERY RIPE BANANA WITH BROWN SKIN (OPTIONAL)
JUICE OF 2 ORANGES
JUICE OF 1 LEMON
MAPLE SYRUP

1   Scoop out passionfruit flesh and blend with optional banana and fruit juice. Add maple syrup to taste.
2   Freeze as above.
3   Alternatively, pour into individual moulds or orange shells and freeze without stirring.

Banana Sticks

5 BANANAS
½ CUP MAPLE SYRUP
1 CUP GROUND LIGHTLY TOASTED NUTS AND SEEDS
½ CUP CAROB POWDER AND/OR DESICCATED COCONUT

1   Peel bananas and cut in half. Thread each one with a bamboo skewer.
2   Dip in maple syrup, roll in nut-sed mixture and then in carob and/or coconut, and freeze.

FRESH FRUIT DESSERTS

Annie's Peaches
Stuffed Ginger Apples
Summer Berries
Apple Pear Walnut Crisp

ANNIE'S PEACHES

1 kg FRESH PEACHES

2 T MAPLE SYRUP

1 x 3 cm CINNAMON STICK

3 – 4 WHOLE CLOVES

2 T BRANDY

1   Peel and seed peaches and cut in half.
2   Place in saucepan with maple syrup, cinnamon and cloves, cover and simmer over medium heat 3 – 4 minutes. (Shake pan occasionally).
3   Remove from heat and add brandy.
4   Peaches will keep for 2 weeks in glass jars in refrigerator.

STUFFED GINGER APPLES

$2/3$ CUP CURRANTS OR SULTANAS

½ CUP *MIRIN*

1½ CUP GROUND ROASTED SUNFLOWER SEEDS

½ t CINNAMON

½ t GROUND CORIANDER

1 T WHITE *MISO*

1 T MINCED GINGER ROOT

1 T MINCED ORANGE RIND

8 BAKING APPLES

$2/3$ CUP *MIRIN*

$2/3$ CUP FRUIT JUICE

SEVERAL T MALTOSE OR BROWN RICE MALT SYRUP (OPTIONAL)

GROUND *KUZU* OR ARROWROOT FLOUR

Forward planning: *Preheat oven to 190°C.*

MACROBIOTICS & BEYOND

1   Soak dried fruit in mirin for 10 minutes. Stir in seeds, cinnamon, coriander, miso, ginger root and orange rind and blend well.

2   Slice 6 mm off tops of apples and remove cores, keeping apple flesh intact at the bottom. Arrange apples in baking dish.

3   Spoon fruit mixture into each cavity.

4   Combine mirin and fruit juice and pour one half around apples.

5   Heat optional maltose or malt syrup and spoon over apples.

6   Bake at 190°C for 30 minutes or until apples are tender. Either bake uncovered, basting frequently with juice in dish, or bake covered, basting once or twice. Remove apples to serving dish.

7   Combine any remaining juice with remaining $2/3$ cup juice-mirin mixture. Thicken with kuzu or arrowroot. (Use 2 t kuzu per cup of liquid.) Pour over apples.

SUMMER BERRIES

¾ CUP BLUEBERRIES OR RASPBERRIES (1 PUNNET)

1 PUNNET STRAWBERRIES

1 T FRESH LIME JUICE

½ CUP MAPLE SYRUP

¼ CUP RUM OR SHERRY

3 T ALMOND OR CASHEW BUTTER

1   Pick over berries and rinse lightly. Hull strawberries and slice thinly.

2   Combine lime juice, maple syrup, rum or sherry and nut butter in sauce-pan. Warm mixture but do not boil it.

3   Toss berries gently with sauce.

4   Serve with poached peaches, cake or ice-cream.

APPLE PEAR WALNUT CRISP

Fruit Mixture

1 kg MIXED APPLES AND PEARS

¼ CUP SOYMILK

4 T TAHINI

½ T VANILLA

1 T FINELY GRATED ORANGE RIND

½ T MINCED GINGER ROOT

1½ t CINNAMON

Topping

¾ CUP CHOPPED WALNUTS
¾ CUP ROLLED OATS
¼ CUP WHOLEWHEAT CAKE OR PASTRY FLOUR
PINCH SEA SALT
⅓ CUP OIL
½ CUP MAPLE SYRUP
¼ CUP *MIRIN*, MARSALA OR SWEET SHERRY

Forward planning: *Preheat oven to 180°C. Oil a gratin or pie dish.*
1 Peel apples and pears and slice thinly.
2 Combine remaining six ingredients and toss fruit slices with the mixture.
3 Spoon apples and pears into oiled pie dish.
Topping
4 Combine the first four ingredients.
5 Beat oil, maple syrup and mirin until thick and creamy. Add to dry mixture to form a fairly dry crumble, adding a little fruit juice or water if necessary.
6 Sprinkle Topping over Fruit Mixture. Press it over top and around edges of dish to seal in fruit.
7 Bake at 180°C for 20 minutes or until fruit is cooked and Topping is crisp and lightly browned.

TARTS, PUFFS AND OTHER SWEET DELIGHTS

Fruit Tart
Blueberry Cream Pie
Sweet Puffs
Walnut Bean Puffs
Oatmeal Cinnamon Puffs
Carob Fudge
Walnut or Almond Balls

FRUIT TART

Pastry

1 CUP ROLLED OATS

1 CUP WHOLEWHEAT CAKE OR PASTRY FLOUR

1 CUP GROUND NUTS OR SEEDS

½ t CINNAMON

PINCH SEA SALT

⅓ – ½ CUP OIL

¼ – ⅓ CUP MAPLE SYRUP

WATER OR FRUIT JUICE AS NEEDED

1 EGG WHITE

Filling

5 T AGAR-AGAR FLAKES

2 CUPS FRUIT JUICE

½ CUP *MIRIN*

2 T MAPLE SYRUP

2 T NUT BUTTER (ALMOND, CASHEW, SESAME, HAZELNUT)

1 T GROUND *KUZU* OR ARROWROOT FLOUR

1 – 2 t VANILLA

FINELY GRATED RIND OF 1 ORANGE OR LEMON

1 WELL-BEATEN EGG YOLK

Topping

FRESH FRUIT IN SEASON

SWEET DELIGHTS

Glaze

½ CUP FRUIT JUICE

1 t GROUND *KUZU* OR ARROWROOT FLOUR

2 t MAPLE SYRUP (OPTIONAL)

1 t RUM, BRANDY OR COGNAC

Forward planning: *Preheat oven to 180°C. Oil a 23 cm pie dish. Pastry can be prepared one day ahead.*

Pastry

1   *Blend oats in blender or food processor until lightly cracked.*

2   *Combine the first five ingredients.*

3   *Beat oil maple syrup until thick and creamy. Add to dry mixture to form a dough and blend until dough begins to leave the sides of the bowl and forms a ball. Add water or fruit juice if necessary to bind the dough.*

4   *Roll out dough on greaseproof paper and invert over oiled pie dish, positioning dough to line dish evenly. Prick pastry with a fork and brush with the egg white which has been broken up with a fork. Bake at 180°C for 15 minutes or until crust is firm and lightly browned.*

5   *Remove from oven and leave to cool.*

Filling

6   *Combine agar-agar and fruit juice in saucepan and bring to the boil. Lower heat, add mirin and optional maple syrup, and simmer until agar-agar dissolves.*

7   *Remove a small amount of the simmering liquid and stir into the nut butter. Add nut butter and kuzu or arrowroot to the saucepan and bring to the boil, stirring continuously.*

8   *Remove from heat, add vanilla, grated rind and beaten egg yolk. Set aside to cool slightly.*

Glaze

9   *Dissolve kuzu or arrowroot in fruit juice in saucepan. Bring to the boil over medium heat, stirring continuously until juice thickens and turns clear. Remove from heat and add rum, brandy or cognac. Set aside to cool slightly.*

To compose tart

10   *Fill cooled pie shell with slightly cooled fruit Filling.*

11   *When Filling is almost set, decorate with fruit in season.*

12   *Spoon Glaze over fruit. Brush any unglazed fruit with Glaze.*

BLUEBERRY CREAM PIE

Pastry

1 CUP ROLLED OATS

½ CUP WHOLEWHEAT CAKE OR PASTRY FLOUR

4 T CAROB FLOUR (ALTERNATIVELY, MAY BE USED IN FILLING)

2 t CINNAMON

PINCH SEA SALT

¼ CUP OIL

¼ CUP MAPLE SYRUP

WATER OR FRUIT JUICE AS NEEDED

Filling

600 g TOFU

2 LARGE OR 3 SMALL EGG YOLKS

½ CUP MAPLE SYRYP

1 T FINELY GRATED LEMON RIND

1 t LEMON JUICE

1 t VANILLA

3 – 4 T GROUND *KUZU* OR ARROWROOT FLOUR

2 LARGE OR 3 SMALL EGG WHITES (AT ROOM TEMPERATURE)

Topping

2 T GROUND *KUZU* OR ARROWROOT FLOUR

1½ CUP FRUIT JUICE

¼ CUP MAPLE SYRUP

4 CUPS BLUEBERRIES (4 PUNNETS)

Forward planning: *Preheat oven to 190°C. Oil a 25 cm springform pan.*

Pastry

1   *Blend oats in blender or food processor until lightly cracked.*

2   *Combine the first six ingredients.*

3   *Beat oil and maple syrup until thick and creamy. Add to dry mixture to form a dough and blend until dough begins to leave the sides of the bowl and form a ball. Add water or fruit juice if necessary to bind the dough.*

4   *Press the dough evenly on the base and sides of an oiled 25 cm springform pan. Prick pastry with a fork and bake at 190°C for 10 – 15 minutes or until crust is firm and lightly browned.*

5   *Remove from oven and leave to cool.*

Filling

6   *Blanch tofu by dropping it into boiling water for 1 minute and drain well.*

7   *Break tofu into chunks and blend with egg yolks, maple syrup, lemon rind and*

SWEET DELIGHTS

juice and vanilla.

8 Fold kuzu or arrowroot flour into mixture.

9 Beat egg whites with a pinch of salt until stiff peaks are formed. Fold carefully into tofu mixture.

10 Spoon Filling into baked crust and bake at 190°C for 30 – 40 minutes or until the centre of Filling is almost firm.

11 Leave to cool in oven with door open.

Topping

12 Dissolve kuzu or arrowroot in fruit juice and maple syrup in saucepan. Bring to the boil over medium heat, stirring until juice thickens and turns clear.

13 Fold in blueberries.

14 When slightly cooled, spoon over Filling.

SWEET PUFFS

Puffs

2 t DRIED YEAST
½ – 1 CUP WARM FRUIT JUICE OR WATER
1 CUP CHICKPEA AND ½ CUP WHOLEWHEAT CAKE OR PASTRY FLOUR, OR
1½ CUPS WHOLEWHEAT CAKE OR PASTRY FLOUR
1 EGG (OPTIONAL)
OIL FOR DEEP FRYING

Glaze

2 CUPS MAPLE SYRUP
2 T LEMON JUICE
½ t CINNAMON
½ t GROUND CARDAMON
CINNAMON
DESICCATED COCONUT (OPTIONAL)

Puffs

1 Dissolve yeast in juice or water and set aside until yeast bubbles.

2 Beat into flour and beat in egg if desired. Beat to form a soft dough that drops from a spoon, adding more juice or water if necessary.

3 Heat oil in wok or pan to deep frying temperature (180° – 190°C) – see p.128 for deep-frying method. Drop teaspoons of batter into oil and deep fry 3 – 4 minutes, turning Puffs as necessary, until puffy. Drain well on rack or absorbent paper.

Glaze

4 Combine maply syrup, lemon juice, cinnamon and cardamon in saucepan and simmer 5 minutes.

MACROBIOTICS & BEYOND

5   Dip Puffs into mixture to coat them.
6   Stack Puffs on a platter, sprinkle with cinnamon and optional coconut and serve immediately.

WALNUT BEAN PUFFS

Filling

1 CUP DRY *ADUKI* BEANS, SOAKED OVERNIGHT IN WATER TO COVER BY AT
   LEAST 5 cm

1 CUP FINELY CHOPPED MIXED DRIED FRUIT

1 CUP GROUND LIGHTLY TOASTED WALNUTS

Pastry

2 CUPS STEAMED SWEET POTATO OR TARO ROOT

2 CUPS SWEET RICE FLOUR

¾ CUP SESAME SEEDS

OIL FOR DEEP FRYING

Forward planning: *Soak aduki beans overnight. Steam sweet potato or taro root.*
Filling

1   Drain aduki beans and cover by at least 5 cm with fresh water in saucepan. Bring beans to the boil, lower heat and simmer uncovered for 20 minutes.

2   Cover beans and simmer 45 – 60 minutes or until soft. Alternatively, pressure cook for 20 minutes.

3   Drain off cooking liquid to leave beans covered by 2.5 cm of liquid. Mix in dried fruit, bring to the boil, lower heat and simmer uncovered until no liquid remains.

4   Blend the mixture until smooth and creamy. Fold in ground walnuts. Leave to cool.
Pastry

5   Mash sweet potato or taro root and blend with sweet rice flour. Knead or blend to a smooth dough, adding a little liquid if necessary.

6   Roll dough into a long log and cut into 32 pieces. Keep dough covered with a damp cloth.

7   Roll each piece into a 5 cm circle. Cup each circle in the hand and place a portion of the Filling in the centre. Gather the dough up around the Filling and pinch to seal at the top.

8   Dip puffs in water and roll in sesame seeds.

9   Heat oil in a wok or pan to deep frying temperature (180° – 190°C) – see p.128 for deep-frying method. Deep fry puffs for 3 – 4 minutes or until golden brown. Drain well on rack or absorbent paper.

10   Serve immediately with lemon or lime slices.
NOTE: Use leftover walnut bean paste for spreads, or thin with stock for soup.

S W E E T   D E L I G H T S

OATMEAL CINNAMON ROLLS

2 t DRIED YEAST

½ CUP WARM FRUIT JUICE OR WATER

1 ½ CUPS SOYMILK OR NUT MILK (see tofu loaf, p. 55)

¼ CUP OIL

¾ CUP ROLLED OATS

¼ MAPLE SYRUP

1 EGG, LIGHTLY BEATEN

PINCH SEA SALT

3½ – 4 CUPS WHOLEWHEAT FLOUR

1 CUP CURRANTS OR SULTANAS

½ t CINNAMON

¼ CUP WHOLEWHEAT BREADCRUMBS OR CAROB FLOUR (OPTIONAL)

MAPLY SYRUP (TO BRUSH ON ROLLS)

Forward planning: *Preheat oven to 180°C.*

1   Dissolve yeast in fruit juice or water and set aside until yeast bubbles.

2   Heat milk and stir in oil. Leave to cool for 10 minutes.

3   Blend oats, maple syrup, beaten egg and sea salt into milk-oil mixture. Stir the mixture into the yeast mixture.

4   Gradually add flour and mix to a soft dough, adding a little liquid if necessary. Knead by hand for 10 minutes. Place dough in oiled bowl, cover and leave to rise until dough is doubled in bulk.

5   Cover dried fruit with boiling water and leave for 10 minutes. Drain well.

6   Punch down dough and roll into a large rectangle. Brush surface with oil.

7   Combine cinnamon with optional breadcrumbs or carob flour and sprinkle over dough, or sprinkly with cinnamon only.

8   Sprinkle fruit over dough, leaving a 2.5 cm border.

9   Roll the dough into a log along the longer side. Pinch edges of dough to seal. Cut into 12 pieces. Arrange pieces, cut-side down, on oiled baking trays, leaving space for dough to rise. Leave to rise uncovered until almost doubled in size.

10   Bake at 180°C for 30 – 40 minutes or until golden brown.

11   Remove from oven and brush with maple syrup immediately.

CAROB FUDGE

4 T AGAR-AGAR FLAKES
½ CUP FRUIT JUICE
½ CUP MAPLE SYRUP
1½ T GROUND *KUZU* OR ARROWROOT FLOUR
½ CUP ROASTED CAROB FLOUR
½ CUP TAHINI
½ CUP CHOPPED WALNUTS
2 T VANILLA

1   Combine agar-agar and fruit juice in saucepan and bring to the boil. Lower heat and simmer until agar-agar dissolves.
2   Add maple syrup, kuzu or arrowroot, carob and tahini, and bring back to the boil. Lower heat and simmer 3 – 4 minutes, stirring continuously, until mixture thickens.
3   Remove from heat and stir in walnuts and vanilla.
4   Pour Fudge into mould 15 cm x 6 cm x 2.5 cm. Leave to cool.
5   Chill and cut into squares.

WALNUT OR ALMOND BALLS

½ CUP FINELY GROUND WALNUTS OR ALMONDS
¼ CUP CHOPPED ROASTED WALNUTS OR ALMONDS
¼ CUP TAHINI OR CASHEW NUT BUTTER
3 – 4 T MAPLE SYRUP
1 T CAROB FLOUR
½ t ROSE WATER OR VANILLA
¼ CUP DESICCATED COCONUT OR TOASTED SESAME SEEDS

1   Combine the first six ingredients and knead together or blend until firm, adding a little liquid if necessary.
2   Roll into a log and divide into walnut-sized pieces. Shape into balls. Roll in coconut or seeds.

CAKES

Apple Walnut Cake
Pear and Pine Nut Supreme Cake
Carrot and Sultana Cake
Julie's Cake
Bo's Sixth Birthday Cake

NOTE: Most of these cake recipes rely on eggs, home-made baking powder and/or yeast for lightness in texture. Because the flour that is recommended has not been pre-sifted, bleached, bromated or stripped of all the bran, it reacts differently with other ingredients. Most of the cakes will not rise 10 cm (3 – 4 in); they will be lower than the normal 'layer cake'. If you would like a higher cake, bake three layers instead of two, or increase the amount of yeast suggested by one half, or double the amount of eggs.

APPLE WALNUT CAKE

1½ CUPS WHOLEWHEAT CAKE OR PASTRY FLOUR
¾ t BICARBONATE OF SODA
2 t CINNAMON
1 CUP GROUND WALNUTS
2 EGGS
¾ CUP MAPLE SYRUP
¾ CUP OIL
1 CUP APPLE SAUCE
2 t VANILLA

Forward planning: *Preheat oven to 190°C. Oil a 23 cm cake pan.*

1   *Combine flour, bicarbonate of soda, cinnamon and walnuts.*

2   *Beat eggs, maple syrup and oil until thick and creamy. Beat in apple sauce and vanilla.*

3   *Fold the wet mixture into the dry one.*

4   *Pour mixture into an oiled 23 cm pan and bake at 190°C for 35 minutes or until cake tester comes out dry.*

MACROBIOTICS & BEYOND

PEAR AND PINE NUT SUPREME CAKE

Pear Topping
2 – 3 RIPE PEARS
6 CLOVES
1 CUP FRUIT JUICE
1 x 2.5 cm CINNAMON STICK
2 T MAPLE SYRUP
¼ CUP BRANDY

Pine Nut Cake
¾ CUP COUSCOUS
1 CUP BOILING WATER (OPTIONAL)
3 T AGAR-AGAR FLAKES
1¾ CUPS FRUIT JUICE
½ T CINNAMON
1¼ CUPS GROUND PINE NUTS

Cake Coating
3 CUPS LIQUID (PEAR COOKING LIQUID AND FRUIT JUICE AS NEEDED)
6 T AGAR-AGAR FLAKES
2 T GROUND *KUZU* OR ARROWROOT FLOUR
3 – 4 t GINGER JUICE (see broccoli cauliflower mousseline, p. 28)
MANDARIN SEGMENTS OR SLICES OF OTHER FRUIT IN SEASON

Forward planning: *Prepare pears. Oil a 25 – 30 cm cake pan, preferably spring-form.*

Pear Topping

1   Peel pears, cut in half and remove cores. Insert one clove in each half.

2   Combine juice, cinnamon stick and maple syrup in a small saucepan and bring to the boil. Immerse the pears in the liquid and simmer 10 minutes or until almost tender. Remove pears and set aside.

3   Add brandy to liquid and use as part of 3 cups liquid required for Cake Coating.

Pine Nut Cake

4   Oil fingers, rub couscous through them, and then steam couscous for 10 minutes. Alternatively, pour boiling water over couscous and leave for 10 minutes.

5   Combine fruit juice and agar-agar in saucepan and bring to the boil. Lower heat and simmer until agar-agar dissolves. Add cinnamon and nuts.

6   Stir the couscous into the mixture and pour into an oiled 25 – 30 cm pan.

Cake Coating

7   Combine juice (including pear liquid) and agar-agar in saucepan and bring to the boil. Lower heat and simmer until agar-agar dissolves. Add kuzu *or arrowroot*

C A K E S

dissolved in a little cold juice and the ginger juice.

8   Spoon Cake Coating over the couscous mixture and leave till almost set.

To complete:

9   Decorate cake with prepared topping, mandarin segments and/or sliced fruit in season, and wait till firm to serve.

CARROT AND SULTANA CAKE

2 CUPS GRATED CARROT

1 CUP SULTANAS

1 t CINNAMON

½ t NUTMEG

¾ CUP FRUIT JUICE

¼ CUP OIL

½ CUP MAPLE SYRUP

1 t VANILLA

2 EGGS YOLKS

1½ CUPS WHOLEWHEAT CAKE OR PASTRY FLOUR

⅔ t CREAM OF TARTAR

⅓ t BICARBONATE OF SODA

⅔ t ARROWROOT

½ CUP GROUND ROLLED OATS

½ CUP CHOPPED WALNUTS

2 EGG WHITES (AT ROOM TEMPERATURE)

Forward planning: *Preheat oven to 180°C. Oil a 23 cm cake pan.*

1   Simmer grated carrot, sultanas, cinnamon and nutmeg in juice for 10 minutes. Cool.

2   Beat oil, maple syrup and vanilla until thick and creamy. Add egg yolks and beat in well.

3   Sift flour with cream of tartar, bicarbonate of soda and arrowroot. Mix with ground rolled oats and fold into egg mixture.

4   Add carrot-juice mixture and walnuts.

5   Beat egg whites with a pinch of salt until stiff peaks are formed and fold carefully into mixture.

6   Pour into oiled 23 cm pan and bake at 180°C for 30 minutes or until cake tester comes out dry.

MACROBIOTICS & BEYOND

JULIE'S CAKE

3½ – 4 CUPS TOASTED GROUND ALMONDS

1 CUP BROWN RICE FLOUR

1 T CINNAMON

¼ CUP CAROB FLOUR

12 EGG YOLKS

¾ CUP MAPLE SYRUP

2 t VANILLA

11 EGG WHITES (AT ROOM TEMPERATURE)

Topping

½ CUP MAPLE SYRUP

1 EGG WHITE

1 t VANILLA

FRESH FRUIT FOR GARNISH

Forward planning: *Preheat oven to 180°C. Oil and flour a 25 cm cake pan, 7.5 cm deep, or two 20 cm pans.*

Cake

1   Combine almonds, flour, cinnamon and carob flour.

2   Beat egg yolks with maple syrup until thick and creamy, adding vanilla slowly.

3   Combine egg yolk mixture with flour mixture.

4   Beat egg whites with a pinch of salt until stiff peaks are formed and fold carefully into mixture, making sure not to deflate egg whites.

5   Spoon mixture into oiled and floured pan(s) and bake in 180°C oven for 30 – 40 minutes or until cake tester comes out dry.

6   Turn off oven and leave cake in oven with door open until cool. Remove from oven and pan.

Topping

7   Heat maple syrup to the 'soft ball' stage (116°C) — use candy thermometer or boil 5 – 8 minutes or until syrup looks like caramel.

8   Beat egg white until stiff peaks are formed, then slowly drip in maple syrup and vanilla.

9   Immediately spread Topping over cake with upward movements to form peaks. Decorate with fresh fruit in season.

C A K E S

BO'S SIXTH BIRTHDAY CAKE

1 CUP WHOLEWHEAT CAKE OR PASTRY FLOUR

½ CUP CAROB FLOUR

3¾ CUPS GROUND NUTS (ALMONDS, PINE NUTS, CASHEWS)

12 EGG YOLKS

1 CUP MAPLE SYRUP

½ CUP OIL

2 CUPS MASHED RIPE BANANAS

12 EGG WHITES (AT ROOM TEMPERATURE)

FRUIT JUICE AS NEEDED

Carob Icing

1 CUP ALMOND OR CASHEW BUTTER

½ CUP MASHED RIPE FRUIT (BANANA, MANGO, PEACH, APRICOT) — OPTIONAL

2 t VANILLA, RUM, BRANDY OR MIRIN

½ t LEMON JUICE

½ CUP CAROB FLOUR

½ CUP MAPLE SYRUP

BOILING FRUIT JUICE AS NEEDED

Forward planning: *Preheat oven to 180°C. Oil and flour a 25 cm cake pan, 7.5 cm deep, or two 20 cm cake pans.*

Cake

1 Combine flour, carob flour and nuts.

2 Beat egg yolks with maple syrup until thick and creamy. Add oil and mashed banana and beat for 3 minutes or until smooth.

3 Combine flour mixture with egg-yolk mixture and set aside.

4 Beat egg whites with a pinch of salt until stiff peaks are formed. Fold whites carefully into the cake mixture. Add fruit juice if necessary to get the right consistency.

5 Spoon mixture into oiled and floured pan(s) and bake 30 – 40 minutes in 180°C oven or until cake tester comes out clean.

6 Turn off oven and leave cake in oven with door open until cool. Remove from pan when ready to ice and serve.

Carob Icing

7 Warm nut butter to room temperature to soften it. Blend with optional fruit, flavouring and lemon juice until smooth and creamy.

8 Beat in carob flour and maple syrup, adding boiling fruit juice as needed until icing is smooth and creamy. (If refrigerating before using, add more boiling fruit juice as needed to bring to desired consistency.)

9 Ice cake and decorate with fresh fruit in season.

COOKIES, BISCUITS AND BARS

Everyone's Favourite Biscuit
Big Spoon Cookies
Nut Rounds
Great Big Ones
Ginger Drops
Five Spice Cookies
Date Nut Bars
Fruit and Nut Squares
Apple Macaroon Slices
Yellow Diamonds

NOTE: When making cookies and biscuits, remove them from the oven before they are browned and fully baked. Otherwise they will become overcooked, as they continue to cook for a few minutes after removal from the oven.

EVERYONE'S FAVOURITE BISCUIT

1 CUP ROLLED OATS
1 CUP GROUND BLANCHED ALMONDS
1 CUP WHOLEWHEAT CAKE OR PASTRY FLOUR
½ t CINNAMON
PINCH SEA SALT
½ CUP MAPLE SYRUP
⅓ – ½ CUP OIL
FRUIT JUICE AS NEEDED
MAPLE SYRUP (TO BRUSH ON BISCUIT)

Forward planning: *Preheat oven to 190°C. Oil a cookie sheet.*
1 Blend oats in blender or food processor until lightly cracked.
2 Combine the first five ingredients.
3 Beat maple syrup and oil until thick and creamy. Add to dry mixture all at once to form a dough, adding fruit juice if necessary.
4 Roll out dough to 6 mm thickness and cut into shapes with a knife or cookie cutters. Place on oiled cookie sheet and bake at 190°C for 15 – 20 minutes or until

COOKIES AND BISCUITS

underside is lightly browned.

5 Remove from oven and brush with maple syrup. Remove to racks and leave to cool.

BIG SPOON COOKIES

¾ CUP GROUND BLANCHED ALMONDS
½ CUP GROUND SUNFLOWER SEEDS
2 CUPS DESICCATED COCONUT
3½ CUPS BROWN RICE FLOUR
2¼ CUPS CURRANTS
3 t CINNAMON
PINCH SEA SALT
4 EGGS (AT ROOM TEMPERATURE)
1 CUP OIL (AT ROOM TEMPERATURE)
½ CUP MAPLE SYRUP
FRUIT JUICE AS NEEDED

Forward planning: *Preheat oven to 190°C. Oil a cookie sheet.*

1 Combine the first seven ingredients.

2 Beat the eggs, oil and maple syrup until thick and creamy. Add to the dry mixture all at once to form a dough, adding fruit juice if necessary.

3 Drop dough from a large spoon onto oiled cookie sheets and bake at 190°C for 10 – 15 minutes or until underside is lightly browned.

4 Remove from oven. Remove to racks and leave to cool.

NUT ROUNDS

1 CUP ROLLED OATS
1 CUP GROUND NUTS (ALMONDS, WALNUTS, PECANS)
1 CUP WHOLEWHEAT CAKE OR PASTRY FLOUR
½ t CINNAMON
PINCH SEA SALT
⅓ CUP MAPLE SYRUP
½ CUP OIL
FRUIT JUICE AS NEEDED

Filling

SUGARLESS FRUIT SPREAD (JAM OR JELLY)

Forward planning: *Preheat oven to 190°C. Oil a cookie sheet.*

1 Blend oats in blender or food processor until lightly cracked.

MACROBIOTICS & BEYOND

2 Combine the first five ingredients.

3 Beat the maple syrup and oil until thick and creamy. Add to the dry ingredients all at once to form a dough, adding fruit juice if necessary.

4 Form into walnut-size balls and place on oiled cookie sheets. Press thumb gently into each ball to make a hole for ½ t fruit spread.

5 Bake at 190°C for 10 – 15 minutes or until underside is lightly browned.

6 Remove from oven. Remove to racks and leave to cool.

GREAT BIG ONES

½ CUP GROUND *KUZU* OR ARROWROOT FLOUR
¾ CUP WHOLEWHEAT CAKE OR PASTRY FLOUR
1 T CINNAMON
PINCH SEA SALT
1 CUP FINELY CHOPPED FRESH APPLES OR PEARS
½ CUP GROUND NUTS OR SEEDS (OPTIONAL)
FINELY GRATED RIND OF 1 LEMON
⅓ CUP OIL
½ – 1 CUP MAPLE SYRUP
FRUIT JUICE AS NEEDED

Forward planning: *Preheat oven to 190°C. Oil a cookie sheet.*

1 Combine the first four ingredients and add fruit, optional nuts or seeds and grated lemon rind.

2 Beat oil and maple syrup until thick and creamy and add all at once to dry mixture. Add fruit juice if necessary to form a batter the consistency of pancake batter.

3 Spoon batter onto oiled cookie sheets and bake at 190°C for 10 – 15 minutes or until crisp.

4 Remove from oven. Remove to racks and leave to cool.

GINGER DROPS

1¾ CUPS WHOLEWHEAT CAKE OR PASTRY FLOUR
¼ CUP BROWN RICE FLOUR OR MAIZEMEAL
1 CUP GROUND WALNUTS
¼ CUP FINELY CHOPPED DRIED FRUIT (OPTIONAL)
2 t GINGER POWDER
1 t CINNAMON

COOKIES AND BISCUITS

½ t GROUND CORIANDER

PINCH SEA SALT

2 EGGS (AT ROOM TEMPERATURE)

½ CUP OIL OR TAHINI

¼ CUP MAPLE SYRUP

BLANCHED ALMONDS

Forward planning: *Preheat oven to 190°C. Oil a cookie sheet.*

1   Combine the first eight ingredients.

2   Beat eggs, oil or tahini and maple syrup until thick and creamy. Mix into dry combination, just until flour is no longer visible.

3   Drop by spoonfuls onto oiled cookie sheets. Press an almond into the centre of each cookie.

4   Bake at 190°C for 10 minutes. Lower heat to 180°C and bake 5 – 10 minutes longer or until underside is lightly browned.

5   Remove from oven. Remove to racks and leave to cool.

FIVE SPICE COOKIE

1½ CUPS WHOLEWHEAT CAKE OR PASTRY FLOUR

1 CUP GROUND TOASTED NUTS OR SEEDS

2 t FIVE SPICE POWDER

1 t CINNAMON

½ t BICARBONATE OF SODA

PINCH SALT

2 EGGS (AT ROOM TEMPERATURE)

½ CUP OIL

½ CUP MAPLE SYRUP

1½ t VANILLA

FRUIT JUICE AS NEEDED

Forward planning: *Preheat oven to 190°C. Oil a cookie sheet.*

1   Combine the first six ingredients.

2   Beat eggs, oil, maple syrup and vanilla until thick and creamy. Add to dry mixture all at once to form a stiff batter, adding fruit juice if necessary.

3   Drop by spoonfuls onto oiled cookie sheets. Bake at 190°C for 10 – 15 minutes or until underside is lightly browned.

4   Remove from oven. Remove to racks and leave to cool.

DATE NUT BARS

Filling

2 CUPS PITTED FINELY CHOPPED DATES

½ CUP FRUIT JUICE

JUICE AND FINELY GRATED RIND OF 1 ORANGE

Crust

1 CUP WHOLEWHEAT CAKE OR PASTRY FLOUR

2 CUPS ROLLED OATS

1 CUP GROUND NUTS

½ T CINNAMON

PINCH SEA SALT

¼ CUP OIL

¼ CUP MAPLE SYRUP

¼ CUP FRUIT JUICE

EXTRA FRUIT JUICE AS NEEDED

Forward planning: *Preheat oven to 180°C. Oil a baking tray with shallow sides. Make Filling.*

1   To make Filling, simmer dates in fruit juice until soft. Mix in orange juice and grated rind to form a smooth purée. Set aside.

2   For the Crust, combine the first five ingredients. Beat oil, maple syrup and fruit juice until thick and creamy. Add all at once to dry mixture to form dough, adding more fruit juice if necessary.

3   Divide the dough in half. Press one half into the oiled tray and cover evenly with the Filling. Break up the remaining dough and sprinkle over the Filling.

4   Bake at 180°C for 20 minutes or until crisp and golden.

5   Remove from oven. Leave to cool in tray. Cut into rectangles.

FRUIT AND NUT SQUARES

1 PEELED AND SEEDED ORANGE

1 CUP GROUND SESAME OR SUNFLOWER SEEDS

1 CUP GROUND NUTS (ALMONDS, WALNUTS, PECANS)

1 CUP FINELY CHOPPED DRIED FRUIT

½ CUP WHOLEWHEAT CAKE OR PASTRY FLOUR

½ CUP ARROWROOT FLOUR

2 t CINNAMON

PINCH SEA SALT

½ CUP MAPLE SYRUP OR AS NEEDED

COOKIES AND BISCUITS

Forward planning: *Preheat oven to 180°C. Oil a baking tray with shallow sides.*
1 *Chop orange and blend with seeds, nuts and fruit.*
2 *Combine flours, cinnamon and sea salt and add to the orange mixture.*
3 *Bind to a dough with maple syrup.*
4 *Press into an oiled baking tray with shallow sides. Cover with foil and bake at 180°C for 15 – 20 minutes. Uncover and bake 15 – 20 minutes longer or until sides begin to pull away from the tray.*
5 *Remove from oven. Leave to cool in tray. Cut into squares.*

APPLE MACAROON SLICES

Crust
1 CUP TOASTED ROLLED OATS
1 CUP WHOLEWHEAT CAKE OR PASTRY FLOUR
2 CUPS DESICCATED COCONUT
½ CUP ROASTED GROUND HAZELNUTS
PINCH SEA SALT
½ CUP OIL
1 CUP FRUIT JUICE OR AS NEEDED
2 t VANILLA
Topping
3 CUPS COOKED APPLE
4 EGG WHITES (AT ROOM TEMPERATURE)
2 CUPS ROASTED DESICCATED COCONUT
1 T ROASTED WHOLEWHEAT CAKE OR PASTRY FLOUR
½ CUP FRUIT JUICE

Forward planning: *Preheat oven to 180°C. Oil a baking tray with shallow sides.*
1 *Blend oats in blender or food processor until lightly cracked.*
2 *Combine the five dry ingredients for the Crust. Rub the oil into the mixture and add juice and vanilla to form a thick batter.*
3 *Spread mixture 2 cm thick onto oiled baking tray. Bake at 180°C for 20 minutes or until cooked.*
4 *Remove from oven and spread Crust evenly with cooked apples.*
5 *Beat egg whites with a pinch of salt to form stiff peaks. Fold coconut and flour in carefully. Stir fruit juice through gently.*
6 *Spread Topping evenly over apples. Bake at 180°C for 20 minutes or until cooked and golden.*
7 *Remove from oven. Leave to cool in tray.*

YELLOW DIAMONDS

⅔ CUP FINELY CHOPPED CURRANTS, SULTANAS OR DATES
FRUIT JUICE TO COVER DRIED FRUIT
1½ CUPS MAIZEMEAL
1¼ CUPS WHOLEWHEAT CAKE OR PASTRY FLOUR
PINCH SEA SALT
¼ CUP DESICCATED COCONUT
FINELY GRATED RIND OF 2 LEMONS OR ORANGES
1 – 2 EGGS (AT ROOM TEMPERATURE)
⅔ CUP OIL
⅓ CUP MAPLE SYRUP
½ CUP CHOPPED NUTS OR SEEDS
1 T RUM OR VANILLA
MAPLE SYRUP (TO BRUSH ON BISCUITS)

Forward planning: *Preheat oven to 180°C. Oil cookie sheets.*
1 Soak dried fruit in lukewarm fruit juice for 10 – 20 minutes. Drain fruit and reserve juice.
2 Sift maizemeal, flour and sea salt into a bowl or onto a flat surface and mix in coconut and grated citrus rind.
3 Beat eggs, oil and maple syrup until thick and creamy. Stir in fruit, nuts or seeds and rum or vanilla. Add all at once to the dry mixture to form a dough, adding fruit juice if necessary.
4 Shape small pieces of dough into oval shapes. Place on oiled cookie sheets and bake at 180°C for 20 – 30 minutes or until underside is lightly browned.
5 Remove from oven and brush with maple syrup. Remove to racks and leave to cool.

BREAKFAST RECIPES

Oat Almond Pikelets
Rolled Pancakes
Spinach Crepes
Potato Pancakes with Poached Eggs
Strawberry Pancakes
Sweet Corn Popovers
Casserole Special
Sunday Loaf
Olive Peasant Bread
Foccacia for Friends
Four Seasons Jam
Tasty Spreads
Soy Spritzers
Congee

OAT ALMOND PIKELETS

2 CUPS ROLLED OATS
½ CUP FINELY GROUND BLANCHED ALMONDS
½ CUP HOT FRUIT JUICE
¾ CUP COLD FRUIT JUICE OR WATER
½ T MAPLE SYRUP
½ T OIL

Forward planning: *Prepare batter the night before.*

1   *Blend oats in blender or food processor until lightly cracked.*

2   *Blend ground almonds and hot fruit juice until thick and creamy. Stir into oats with cold juice or water, maple syrup and oil, to make a smooth pancake batter.*

3   *Leave batter to stand overnight at room temperature. When ready to use, thin with water or juice if necessary.*

4   *Heat skillet and oil lightly with paper towel. Spoon in batter, about 2 T for each pikelet. Cook until golden brown on each side.*

5   *Serve with fruit topping.*

ROLLED PANCAKES

SHEETS *NORI* SEA VEGETABLE

2 CUPS WHOLEWHEAT CAKE OR PASTRY FLOUR

2 EGGS

WARM WATER

SEA SALT

1   Toast each nori sheet, shiny side down, over low heat until it turns green. Set aside.

2   Beat flour and eggs together. Slowly add warm water to make a smooth pancake batter. Add sea salt to taste.

3   Leave batter to stand 15 minutes at room temperature.

4   Heat skillet and oil lightly with paper towel. Spoon in enough batter to cover bottom of skillet. Cook pancake on each side until lightly browned.

5   Place nori sheet on each pancake and roll up.

6   Serve with sweet or savoury sauce.

SPINACH CREPES

1 CUP WHOLEWHEAT CAKE OR PASTRY FLOUR

1½ CUP SOYMILK, NUTMILK (see tofu loaf, p. 55) OR COCONUT MILK

2 EGGS

2 T OIL

SEA SALT TO TASTE

Filling

2 CUPS FINELY CHOPPED COOKED SPINACH

½ CUP SAUTÉED, THINLY SLICED MUSHROOMS

½ CUP FINELY CHOPPED NUTS

3 – 4 T ALMOND NUT BUTTER

½ – 1 T *MISO* OR SEA SALT TO TASTE

Sauce

1 CUP SLICED SPRING ONIONS OR SHALLOTS

4 T OIL

4 T *MIRIN* OR SWEET SHERRY

1 T BROWN RICE VINEGAR

3 T BROWN RICE FLOUR, CHICKPEA FLOUR *(BESAN)* OR BARLEY FLOUR

2½ – 3 CUPS WARM SOYMILK, NUTMILK (see tofu loaf, p. 55) OR COCONUT MILK

B R E A K F A S T   R E C I P E S

1 T DRIED BASIL OR OREGANO

SHOYU OR *TAMARI* TO TASTE

SPROUTS FOR GARNISH

Forward planning: *Crepe batter, Filling and Sauce may be prepared the day before.*

Crepe batter

  1   Combine all crepe ingredients and blend quickly for about 30 seconds.

  2   Leave to stand overnight, or for at least 30 minutes, at room temperature.

Filling

  3   Combine spinach, mushrooms and nuts with nut butter and miso or sea salt.

Sauce

  4   Heat skillet, add 2 T oil and sauté spring onions or shallots until transparent and tender.

  5   Stir in mirin or sherry or vinegar, and simmer until reduced by half. Set aside.

  6   Heat another skillet, add 2 T oil, and blend in flour until it is completely coated with oil and smells cooked.

  7   Slowly add warm milk (soy, nut or coconut), stirring continously until Sauce has thickened and comes to the boil. Add more milk if necessary.

  8   Add herbs, lower heat, cover and simmer 10 minutes.

  9   Add shoyu or tamari and bring to the boil.

  10   Stir onion mixture into Sauce and set aside.

To prepare crepes

  11   Thin out batter with milk (soy, nut or coconut) if necessary. Batter should be of pouring consistency.

  12   Heat crepe pan or skillet and oil lightly with paper towel. Ladle some batter into pan and tilt quickly to coat pan bottom with a thin coating of batter. Pour excess back into bowl.

  13   Cook crepes on each side until lightly browned. Remove to a warm plate.

  14   Mix 1 – 2 T of Sauce into spinach Filling. Place a few spoons of filling in each crepe, roll up and cover with a few spoons of Sauce.

  15   To serve, garnish with sprouts.

MACROBIOTICS & BEYOND

POTATO PANCAKES WITH POACHED EGGS

500 g POTATOES, PEELED AND GRATED OR FINELY CHOPPED

½ CUP GRATED ONION OR SHALLOTS

1 – 2 T FRESHLY GRATED WHOLEMEAL BREADCRUMBS

1½ T WHOLEWHEAT FLOUR, GROUND *KUZU* OR ARROWROOT FLOUR

SEA SALT TO TASTE

FRESHLY GROUND BLACK PEPPER OR JAPANESE SEVEN SPICE CHILI PEPPER
TO TASTE

SEVERAL T OIL

6 EGGS

Forward planning: *Preheat oven to 150°C.*

1   *Combine first six ingredients in large bowl. Divide into six even portions.*

2   *Heat skillet, add 2 T oil, and place one portion of mixture in skillet. Flatten into a pancake until lightly browned on each side. Keep warm in 150°C oven.*

3   *Cook remaining pancakes in the same way and keep warm.*

4   *Poach eggs, remove from water with slotted spoon and pat dry.*

5   *Place a pancake on each plate and top with a poached egg.*

STRAWBERRY PANCAKES

Topping

2 PUNNETS STRAWBERRIES

Filling

170 g TOFU

1 CUP LIGHTLY TOASTED PINE NUTS

MAPLE SYRUP TO TASTE

FRUIT JUICE AS NEEDED

Pancakes

¾ CUP PLAIN YOGHURT

2 EGGS

2 T OIL

4 – 5 T FRUIT JUICE

1 CUP WHOLEWHEAT CAKE OR PASTRY FLOUR

SEA SALT TO TASTE

Forward planning: *Pancake batter and Filling may be prepared the day before.*

1   *Wash, hull, dry and slice strawberries. Set aside.*

2   *Blanch tofu by dropping into boiling water for 1 minute and draining well. Blend*

112

BREAKFAST RECIPES

with pine nuts and maple syrup until smooth, adding fruit juice if necessary. Set aside.

3   Blend yoghurt, eggs, oil and fruit juice until creamy. Stir in flour and sea salt to make a smooth pancake batter.

4   Leave to stand at room temperature for at least 30 minutes.

5   Heat crepe pan or skillet, oil lightly with paper towel and ladle some batter into pan. Cook on each side until lightly browned.

6   Place first pancake on plate and top with some Filling and sliced strawberries. Repeat with each pancake. Top with strawberries.

SWEET CORN POPOVERS

⅓ CUP FRESH SWEET CORN KERNELS

⅓ CUP FRUIT JUICE OR WATER

2 EGGS

½ CUP SOYMILK

1 T OIL

SEA SALT TO TASTE

1 CUP WHOLEWHEAT FLOUR

Forward planning: *Preheat oven to 200°C. Oil 6 large or 12 small cupcake or muffin tins.*

1   Blend corn kernels and juice or water until kernels are finely chopped. Strain liquid into measuring cup to measure ½ cup, adding more juice or water if necessary. Reserve chopped kernels separately.

2   Blend corn liquid with eggs, soymilk, oil and sea salt. Whisk flour into mixture to make a smooth batter. Stir in chopped kernels.

3   Place oiled cupcake or muffin tins on baking sheet and heat in oven until very hot.

4   Remove from oven and IMMEDIATELY ladle batter into each hot cup.

5   Place in oven, reduce temperature to 190°C and bake for 20 minutes or until popovers are firm and browned.

6   Remove from oven and with the tip of a sharp knife slit each popover just above the rim of the cup.

7   Remove popovers from cups carefully and place on their sides on the baking sheet.

8   Place in oven and bake for 5 minutes or until crisp and dry. Serve immediately.

MACROBIOTICS & BEYOND

CASSEROLE SPECIAL

1½ SLICES WHOLEMEAL BREAD
1 CUP SOYMILK
¼ CUP OIL
½ CUP FINELY CHOPPED SHALLOTS
1 CUP FINELY SLICED MUSHROOMS
12 EGGS
¼ CUP FINELY CHOPPED CORIANDER LEAVES
¼ CUP FINELY CHOPPED PARSLEY LEAVES
SEA SALT, *SHOYU* OR *TAMARI*
FRESHLY GROUND BLACK PEPPER
⅓ CUP WATER
325 g FINELY GRATED *MOCHI* (SWEET BROWN RICE CAKES), RENNET-FREE, OR BIO-DYNAMIC HARD CHEESE

Forward planning: *May be prepared up to 12 hours in advance to baking stage. Cover and refrigerate. Bring to room temperature before baking. Preheat oven to 190°C. Oil shallow 6-cup baking dish.*

1   Remove crusts from bread and grate into breadcrumbs. Combine crumbs with soymilk and soak for 5 minutes.

2   Heat skillet, add oil and sauté shallots until transparent and soft. Add mushrooms and sauté until soft. Set aside.

3   Blend eggs well with breadcrumb mixture, coriander, parsley, salt and pepper. Transfer to large bowl and stir in water.

4   Heat mushroom mixture over medium heat and stir in egg mixture. Cook 4 – 5 minutes, stirring until eggs form very soft curds but are not completely set.

5   Immediately spread half egg-mushroom mixture into oiled baking dish. Cover with half mochi or cheese. Repeat layering.

6   Bake casserole in 190°C oven, 15 – 20 minutes or until puffed and lightly browned. Serve immediately.

SUNDAY LOAF

1 PACKAGE (2¼ t) DRIED YEAST
⅓ CUP WARM (40 – 50°C) WATER OR FRUIT JUICE
¼ CUP MAPLE SYRUP
3¼ CUPS WHOLEWHEAT FLOUR
¼ CUP CRACKED WHEAT
SEA SALT TO TASTE
¼ CUP OIL

BREAKFAST RECIPES

1 CUP WATER	
1 CUP SUNFLOWER SEEDS	
½ CUP PUMPKIN SEEDS	
2 T SESAME SEEDS	
2 T POPPY SEEDS	

Forward planning: *Preheat oven to 190°C. Oil baking sheet.*

1   *Combine yeast with warm water or fruit juice and maple syrup, and stir to dissolve. Set aside until yeast has foamed.*

2   *Combine flour, cracked wheat and sea salt.*

3   *Combine oil and water with yeast mixture. Blend into flour mixture to form a dough.*

4   *Knead dough by hand or in food processor until smooth and elastic. Add flour or water if dough is too sticky or too dry.*

5   *Shape dough into a ball and place in a lightly oiled bowl. Lightly oil the top of the dough. Cover bowl and leave dough to rise in a warm place for 1 – 1 ½ hours or until doubles in bulk.*

6   *Punch dough down and knead in all seeds except 2 T pumpkin seeds.*

7   *Divide dough in half and shape each half into a round loaf.*

8   *Place loaves on oiled baking sheet and set aside to rise in a warm place for 1 – 1 ½ hours or until almost doubled in size.*

9   *Coarsely chop remaining 2 T pumpkin seeds and sprinkle over loaves.*

10   *Bake loaves in 190°C oven for 35 minutes or until lightly browned and sounding hollow when tapped.*

11   *Remove from oven and baking sheet then cool on rack.*

OLIVE PEASANT BREAD

1 PACKAGE (2¼ t) DRIED YEAST
1 CUP WARM (40 – 45°C) WATER OR FRUIT JUICE
1 EGG
1 T OIL
1 T FINELY CHOPPED BASIL LEAVES OR ½ t DRIED
1 T FINELY CHOPPED OREGANO LEAVES OR ¾ t DRIED
SEA SALT TO TASTE
1 T MAPLE SYRUP (OPTIONAL)
1¼ CUPS PITTED, COARSELY CHOPPED BLACK OLIVES
3½ – 4 CUPS WHOLEWHEAT FLOUR
1 EGG, BEATEN
POPPY OR SESAME SEEDS

Forward planning: *Preheat oven to 180°C. Oil baking sheet.*

1 Combine yeast with warm water or juice and stir to dissolve. Set aside until yeast has foamed.

2 Blend egg, oil, herbs, sea salt, optional maple syrup, olives and flour into yeast mixture to form a dough.

3 Knead dough by hand or in food processor until smooth and elastic. Add more flour or water if dough is too sticky or too dry.

4 Shape dough into a ball and place in a lightly oiled bowl. Cover bowl and leave dough to rise in a warm place 1 – 1½ hours or until doubled in bulk.

5 Punch dough down and form into a round loaf. Place on lightly oiled baking sheet and set aside to rise in a warm place for 1 – 1½ hours or until almost doubled in size.

6 Brush loaf with beaten egg and top with poppy or sesame seeds.

7 Bake loaf in 180°C oven for 30 – 40 minutes or until lightly browned and sounding hollow when tapped.

8 Remove from oven and baking sheet then cool on rack.

JANET'S FOCCACIA FOR FRIENDS

1 PACKAGE (2¼ t) DRIED YEAST
½ CUP WARM (40 – 45°C) WATER
2½ CUPS WHOLEWHEAT FLOUR OR MIXTURE OF WHOLEWHEAT AND UNBLEACHED WHITE FLOUR
½ CUP BUCKWHEAT FLOUR
¼ CUP OLIVE OIL
¼ CUP WATER
2 t SEA SALT
1½ t FRESH OR 2 t DRIED FINELY CHOPPED ROSEMARY
1 T OLIVE OIL

Forward planning: *Preheat oven to 200°C. Place baking stone on top oven rack, or lightly oil baking sheet.*

1 Combine yeast with warm water and stir to dissolve. Set aside until yeast has foamed.

2 Combine flours.

3 Combine yeast mixture with 1½ cups flour and knead by hand or in food processor until smooth and elastic. Add flour or water if dough is too sticky or too dry.

4 Shape dough into a ball and place in a lightly floured bowl. Cover bowl and leave dough to rise in a warm place for 3 hours or until doubled in bulk.

5 Punch dough down and knead in remaining 1½ cups flour, olive oil, water and

B R E A K F A S T R E C I P E S

sea salt. Continue kneading by hand or in food processor until dough is smooth and elastic. Knead in chopped rosemary by hand, making sure it is distributed evenly through dough.

6 Repeat Step 4.

7 Roll dough into a disk 1.5 – 2 cm thick. Dimple the surface using your fingertips. Dribble the T of oil over the surface.

8 Transfer the dough to the heated baking stone on a floured sheet of thick cardboard, or place in oven on oiled baking sheet. Bake foccacia in 200°C oven for 20 – 25 minutes or until lightly browned and sounding hollow when tapped.

9 Remove from oven and cool on rack. Serve while still warm, if possible.

FOUR SEASONS JAM

5 CUPS FINELY CHOPPED SEASONAL FRESH FRUIT
1 CUP FINELY CHOPPED DRIED FRUIT
FRUIT JUICE OR HALF-JUICE/HALF-WATER TO COVER FRUIT
2 t CINNAMON OR CORIANDER POWDER
2 T *NATTO MISO* OR WHITE *MISO*, OR PINCH OF SEA SALT
3 T GROUND *KUZU* OR ARROWROOT FLOUR

1 Cover fruits with juice in saucepan, add spice and bring to the boil. Cover and simmmer 10 minutes or until fruit is soft.

2 Dissolve miso or sea salt in a little hot juice from the saucepan.

3 Dissolve kuzu or arrowroot in a little cold water, add to the fruit and stir until jam has thickened.

4 Remove from heat, and stir in dissolved miso or sea salt.

5 Spoon into sterilised glass jars and keep in refrigerator for up to 1 month.

NOTE: In winter, smash a piece of fresh ginger root with a heavy knife blade and simmer with the fruit mixture. Remove before using jam.

TASTY SPREADS

Sunshine Spread

½ CUP ALMOND BUTTER
2 – 4 T *MISO*, DEPENDING ON *MISO* TYPE
¼ CUP GRATED APPLE OR OTHER FRUIT IN SEASON
FEW T LEMON JUICE OR OTHER FRUIT JUICE
1 t FINELY GRATED LEMON OR ORANGE RIND (IF NOT USING LEMON JUICE)

1 Combine almond butter, miso and grated fruit.

2 Bring juice almost to boil and blend into mixture until smooth and creamy. Add rind if necessary.

3 Use as spread for bread, toast, waffles or pancakes.

ONION BUTTER

½ CUP OIL

15 CUPS THINLY SLICED ONION

½ CUP *SHOYU* OR *TAMARI*

1½ – 2 CUPS WATER

1 Heat large deep saucepan or wok, add oil and sauté onions until transparent and soft.

2 Combine shoyu or tamari and water, and pour over onions. Bring to the boil, cover and simmer 20 minutes.

3 Remove cover and reduce liquid until none remains.

4 If mixture is not creamy, add 1 cup water and reduce liquid again. Repeat until mixture is smooth and creamy.

5 Use as spead for bread or as sauce for noodles. If too sweet, adjust taste with miso or sea salt.

HAZELNUT MISO SPREAD

1 CUP SKINNED HAZELNUTS

¼ CUP WATER OR FRUIT JUICE

1 – 2 T WHITE *MISO* OR OTHER *MISO* TO TASTE

1 t FINELY GRATED ORANGE RIND

¼ CUP DICED SHALLOTS OR FINELY CHOPPED PARSLEY OR CORIANDER LEAVES

1 Toast hazelnuts if not already toasted, and grind finely.

2 Combine remaining ingredients and blend with nuts until smooth and creamy. Use a little more liquid if necessary.

RAINBOW SPREAD

450 g TOFU

1 T MAPLE SYRUP

1 T COARSE GRAIN PREPARED MUSTARD

2 – 3 t DRIED BASIL OR OREGANO

½ CUP OIL OR CASHEW NUT BUTTER

BREAKFAST RECIPES

1 T BROWN RICE VINEGAR OR LEMON JUICE

2 t GINGER JUICE (see p. 127)

SEA SALT TO TASTE

STOCK OR HOT WATER AS NEEDED

1 CUP MINCED UNCOOKED VEGETABLES

1   Blanch tofu by dropping into boiling water for 1 minute and draining well.

2   Break tofu into chunks and blend until smooth and creamy. Blend in the remaining ingredients except the minced vegetables, using a little stock or hot water if necessary to make a smooth spread.

3   Stir in minced vegetables.

SOY SPRITZERS

½ CUP FLAVOURED SOYMILK OR NUT MILK (see tofu loaf, p. 55)

⅓ – ½ CUP FRUIT JUICE

½ CUP CARBONATED FRUIT JUICE, OR COMBINATION OF FRUIT JUICE (⅔) AND CARBONATED MINERAL WATER (½)

Blend ingredients together.

Strawberry spritzer
Blend together strawberry soymilk, strawberry juice and carbonated cherry juice.

Cherry Carob Delight
Blend together carob soymilk, cherry juice and carbonated apple juice

Vanilla Cola
Blend together vanilla soymilk, cherry juice and cola carbonated pear juice

CONGEE

1 CUP BROWN RICE

5 – 6 CUPS WATER

1   Combine rice and water in a heavy pot.

2   Turn burner to lowest possible heat, cover pot and simmer congee 4 – 6 hours.
Makes 6 – 7 cups congee.

Any of the following ingredients may be added, according to needs:

⅓ – ½ CUP ADUKI BEANS

½ CUP APRICOT KERNELS

2 CUPS CHOPPED CARROTS

2 CUPS CHOPPED CELERY

½ CUP DRIED CHESTNUTS

½ CUP DRIED DATES AND SEVERAL SLICES BRUISED GINGER ROOT
1 - 2 t DRIED GINGER POWDER
1 - 2 t FENNEL SEEDS
2 CUPS CHOPPED LEEKS
½ CUP DRIED *MUNG* BEANS
1 CUP PINE NUTS
2 CUPS CHOPPED RADISH (RED OR WHITE)
2 CUPS CHOPPED SPINACH
2 CUPS CHOPPED TARO ROOT
½ CUP WHEAT BERRIES

BEVERAGES

Berry Soymilk Shake
Apple, Pear and Lemon Smoothie
Daniel's Winter Warmer
Spiced Tea
Hot Orange Tea

BERRY SOYMILK SHAKE

1 CUP BERRIES (STRAWBERRIES, BLUEBERRIES OR RASPBERRIES)
1 t FINELY GRATED ORANGE RIND
1 t GROUND CORIANDER
2 t TAHINI OR OTHER NUT BUTTER
2 CUPS SOYMILK (OR NUTMILK OR OTHER MILK)
¼ – ⅓ CUP MAPLE SYRUP OR OTHER SWEETNER

Blend all the ingredients together.

APPLE, PEAR AND LEMON SMOOTHIE

1 CUP ALMOND MILK (see tofu loaf, p. 55) OR CASHEW MILK OR COCONUT MILK
1 CUP FRUIT JUICE
½ CUP CHILLED GRATED APPLES
1 CUP CHILLED CHOPPED PEARS
1 t CINNAMON
1 t GROUND GINGER
1 t LEMON OR LIME RIND
PINCH SEA SALT (OPTIONAL)

Blend all the ingredients together.

MACROBIOTICS & BEYOND

DANIEL'S WINTER WARMER

6 CUPS FRUIT JUICE (I PREFER APPLE-PEAR JUICE)

3 – 4 CINNAMON STICKS

SEVERAL WHOLE CLOVES

½ t GRATED NUTMEG

3 SLICES BRUISED GINGER ROOT

3 SLICES DRIED LICORICE ROOT*

BRANDY TO TASTE

Combine the juice, cinnamon, cloves, nutmeg, ginger root and licorice root in a saucepan and simmer 20 minutes. Pour brandy into glasses and top with brew.
* Available in Chinese Herbal shops.

SPICED TEA

2 STRIPS LEMON RIND

6 WHOLE CLOVES

5 cm PIECE OF CINNAMON BARK

3 T TEA LEAVES OR TWIGS

LEMON SLICES

Combine the rind, cloves and cinnamon with 5 cups water and bring to the boil. Simmer the mixture for 10 minutes, then return it to the boil. Pour the mixture over the tea in a teapot and set aside to steep 4 – 5 minutes. Strain and serve with lemon slices.

HOT ORANGE TEA

¹/₃ CUP FRESHLY SQUEEZED ORANGE JUICE

4 t TEA LEAVES

LEMON SLICES

In a small heat-proof pitcher, combine the juice and 1 cup boiling water. Pour the mixture over the tea leaves in a teapot, and set aside to steep for 3 – 4 minutes. Add another cup boiling water and set aside for another 3 – 4 minutes. Strain and serve with the lemon slices.

STOCKS AND STANDARD MARINADE

Dashi Stock
Chicken Stock
'Anything Goes' Stock
Basic White Fish Stock
Standard Marinade

DASHI STOCK

Good for soups, boiled dishes, dressings and sauces.

10 – 15 cm (4 x 6 inch) PIECE *KOMBU* SEA VEGETABLE

2½ CUPS WATER

⅔ CUP DRIED *BONITO* FISH FLAKES (OPTIONAL)

1   Wipe the kombu with a dry cloth and make 2 – 3 perpendicular cuts. Place the water in a saucepan, add the kombu and bring ALMOST to the boil.

2   Just before the water starts to boil, remove the kombu. If you let the kombu boil it can become cloudy and have a bitter taste.

3   When the water boils, add 1 cup cold water and the optional bonito flakes, and bring to the boil for about 10 seconds. Remove from the heat.

4   Skim off any residue that has collected on top and set aside for 3 minutes, or until the flakes settle to the bottom.

5   Place a colander, which has been lined with cheesecloth, over a bowl and pour the stock through. DO NOT SQUEEZE THE CLOTH.

6   To store: add a pinch of sea salt and refrigerate in a glass or ceramic bowl for 2 – 3 days. Makes 2½ cups stock.

Re-using the ingredients:

7   Place the used bonito flakes in a skillet and cook stirring constantly until they are dry. Add 1 t toasted sesame seeds and sea salt to taste.

8   Use on top of pasta, grains or salads.

PORRIDGE STOCK

Cook porridge and if it sticks to the bottom of the saucepan, remove all the porridge, add cold water to the saucepan and bring to the boil.

Cover and simmer 15-20 minutes. Use this water for stock:

WHOLE GRAIN STOCK

Follow the instructions for porridge stock, using the bottom of rice, oats, wheat,

MACROBIOTICS & BEYOND

barley, etc.
NOODLE WATER STOCK
Save the cooking water after preparing noodles. Use as a stock, diluted.

CHICKEN STOCK

1¼ kg ROASTING CHICKEN, CUT INTO 5 cm PIECES THROUGH THE BONE

10 CUPS WATER

¼ CUP DRY RICE WINE

3 SLICES GINGER ROOT, SMASHED WITH THE FLAT SIDE OF A KNIFE

1 Blanch the cut chicken pieces in boiling water for 1 minute.
2 Rinse them in cold water and drain well.
3 Place the chicken pieces, water, rice wine and ginger root in a large pot.
4 Bring to the boil, lower heat and simmer uncovered 1½ – 2 hours, occasionally skimming off any impurities that rise to the surface.
5 Strain the broth through cheesecloth or a fine colander. Save the chicken pieces for another use.
6 This stock will keep refrigerated in a glass or porcelain container for 1 week. (May be frozen.)
Makes 6 cups of stock.

'ANYTHING GOES' STOCK

1 Use any ingredients that would otherwise have been thrown away: e.g. onion skins, celery tops, chicken backs and necks, fish heads (from white-meat fish only), prawn peelings, crab claws or bodies, turkey necks — the list is endless.
2 Place them in a large stock pot with some carrots and onions and ginger root slices, cover with water and bring to the boil.
3 Skim off any foam or impurities that rise to the surface, reduce heat to low and simmer for a couple of hours, occasionally skimming the surface.
4 Cool and refrigerate. Skim off fat before using.

STOCKS AND STANDARD MARINADE

BASIC WHITE FISH STOCK

Before using this stock for a sauce or soup, bring it to the boil and reduce it to intensify the flavour. Add sea salt only after reducing the stock and combining it with other ingredients.

2¼ Kg FISH BONES (INCLUDING HEADS), RINSED, DRIED AND CUT INTO 7 cm PIECES (WHITE MEAT FISH HEADS ONLY)

2 T OIL

1 LEEK, WHITE PART ONLY, SLICED THINLY

1 SMALL CARROT, SLICED THINLY

1 SMALL CELERY STALK (WITH LEAVES), SLICED THINLY

10 PARSLEY SPRIGS, WITH STEMS

6 FRESH THYME SPRIGS OR 2 t DRIED THYME, CRUMBLED

6 WHITE PEPPERCORNS, COARSELY CRUSHED

3 STRIPS LEMON PEEL (EACH 3 cm)

2 CUPS RICE WINE (DRY)

5 CUPS COLD WATER

1   *Discard any feathery red gills from fish heads if necessary.*
2   *Heat skillet and add oil, fish bones and the next five ingredients.*
3   *Cover and cook, stirring occasionally, until vegetables are transparent.*
4   *Add peppercorns and lemon peel.*
5   *Add wine and enough water to just cover the ingredients.*
6   *Bring mixture slowly to simmering point.*
7   *Partially cover pan and reduce heat until liquid is just moving. (DO NOT BOIL OR STOCK WILL BE CLOUDY.)*
8   *Cook, skimming foam from surface as necessary, until stock is richly flavoured (about 30 minutes).*
9   *Line a fine sieve or strainer with several pieces of dampened muslin and set over a large bowl.*
10   *Strain stock into bowl, pressing down lightly on fish and vegetables with the back of a spoon to extract as much liquid as possible.*
11   *Cool and chill.*
12   *Discard the fat that accumulates on the top.*
13   *Store in the refrigerator and reboil every 3 days to prevent spoilage.*
Makes 4 cups of stock.

STANDARD MARINADE *(FOR FISH, POULTRY AND TOFU OR TEMPEH)*

1 t EACH OF:

DRY ORANGE PEEL (warm, pungent and bitter, affects the spleen and lungs)

CLOVES (warm, pungent, affects the spleen, kidneys and stomach)

CINNAMON BARK (hot, pungent and sweet, affects the kidneys and liver)

STAR ANISE (warm, sweet and pungent, affects the kidneys and spleen)

BLACK PEPPER (hot, pungent, affects the large intestine and stomach)

NUTMEG (warm, pungent, affects the spleen and large intestine)

SPRING ONION — WHITE BULBS (warm, pungent, affects the stomach and lungs)

RED CHILI (hot, pungent, affects the heart and spleen)

LICORICE (neutral, sweet, affects the spleen, stomach and lungs)

FENNEL (warm, pungent, affects the kidneys, stomach and bladder)

2 CUPS WATER

½ CUP RICE WINE

SHOYU OR *TAMARI* TO TASTE

2 – 3 T BROWN RICE MALT SYRUP OR MALTOSE

1 Wrap the first ten ingredients in a piece of muslin or cheesecloth.

2 Place in saucepan. Add the water, wine, shoyu and sweetener to the saucepan and bring to the boil. Cover and simmer 10 – 15 minutes. Marinate the food of your choice in the sauce for a few hours or simmer the food in the sauce until cooked. Use the leftover marinade for other foods or discard. (DO NOT DRINK.)

GINGER JUICE

(as required for Broccoli Cauliflower Mousseline, and other recipes as indicated)

1 Peeling the ginger
The skin of a ginger root is generally quite rough, except when you get a young ginger root just after it has been harvested. Use the edge of a spoon to scrape away the skin, instead of a knife, to avoid waste.

2 Grating the ginger root
Hold the ginger firmly and grate it in the same direction as the lines that circle the root. In this way the long fibres will stay on the root.

3 Ginger juice
Place the grated ginger root in a small strainer or a damp piece of cheesecloth, and using your fingertips press down firmly on the ginger root, wringing out as much of the juice as possible. Keep a bowl or cup underneath to catch the juice.

DEEP-FRYING

(This method is required for several recipes throughout the book, as indicated.)

Deep-fried foods are light and crisp without a trace of oiliness, providing they are cooked as quickly as possible. In this way the freshness, flavour and nutrition of the foods are preserved.

The secret of perfect deep-frying also lies in the oil used. Pure safflower or corn oil with just a touch of sesame oil added for flavour gives the best results. The oil must be kept at a high and even temperature. You can check this with the following test: Place a wooden spoon or cooking chopstick in the centre of the oil; at 170°C (340°F) at the usual deep-frying temperature, the oil will bubble slightly around the wooden object. Another test is to drop a tiny piece of bread into the hot oil: at 170°C it will sink slightly, then rise quickly to the surface; if it sizzles on the surface of the oil without sinking, the oil temperature is too hot; if it sinks to the bottom and does not rise, the oil is too cold.

Always deep-fry in at least 10 cm of oil, and don't overload the oil. Deep-fry in a small saucepan fitted with a rack so that the oil from the cooked foods can drain back into the pan. Skim the oil after each use; cool it and strain it into a glass jar. Keep it refrigerated and it will be fresh enough to use one or two more times.

Drain deep-fried foods on absorbent paper and serve immediately. If there is any leftover food, re-heat it or serve it in hot soups. Eating cold fried foods is not good for digestion.

A WORD ON RICE — STORING, PREPARING AND COOKING

Rice, one of the most popular grains, has been used as a staple food throughout the world for thousands of years. Mainly used in Asian countries in the past, rice is today finding a home in the West. Brown rice, in particular, is becoming increasingly popular as people look towards a healthier and more sustaining diet.

Brown rice is not only easy to cook and store, but it is also very economical. It can provide you with lots of energy for the day, without being as fattening as white rice. Rice is filled with vitamin B1, B2, and niacin, and when digested it is transformed into amino acids which create nourishment for the muscles, hair, eyes, skin, heart, lungs, brain and blood vessels.

Storing Uncooked Rice

If there is excess humidity or excess heat, in time the rice could sprout or alter its starch structure. Keep the bag or other container tightly closed, and in warmer climates I suggest that you store the grain in the refrigerator. It would be wise to check periodically for undesirable insects as they have a habit of liking to live in wholefoods, especially brown rice and other grains. If you do find bugs in your rice, don't throw it out; just sift out the nests and wash the rice well, as the bugs will float up to the top of the water. This may seem strange at first, but would you throw out a head of lettuce if you found a worm on it? The harmful things are insecticides which leaves residues, not bugs!

Preparing Rice

Most white rice is coated with glucose or talc, so it is necessary to wash the rice several times before cooking. When you buy organic or bio-dynamic rice it is not necessary to wash the rice at all. In fact washing the rice would only remove some of the micronutrients and minerals from the bran.

Try pre-soaking brown rice and boiling it in the soaking liquid. This will shorten the cooking time by 10 minutes and bring out more flavour. Soaking also softens the bran coats, releasing minerals into the water and making the rice sweeter and more digestible.

Cooking Brown Rice

Using a pressure cooker

One cup of rice yields about two to three servings. Just before cooking rinse the rice if it is not organic or bio-dynamically grown. Drain the rice in a colander. Place it in a pressure cooker and add water until the water level comes up to the first horizontal line in your index finger.

Add a pinch of sea salt, attach the lid and place over high heat. When the pressure cooker indicates that it has reached full pressure, reduce the heat to low and cook another 30 – 40 minutes. Remove from the heat and let it stand for 15 minutes. Remove the lid and stir the rice FROM TOP TO BOTTOM, mixing well.

Stainless steel saucepan
Wash the rice if necessary (see above) and soak it for a few hours before cooking, using 1.4 – 1.5 parts of water to 1 part rice for a dry consistency, or 2 parts water to 1 part rice for a more moist consistency. This is relative to the type of rice you use (short, medium or long grain) and the season or particular weather that day (the more moist the day the less water is needed), as well as the type of pot you use. Place the saucepan over a medium heat and when the water comes to the boil, reduce heat, cover and simmer 40 – 45 minutes. Remove from heat and set aside for 10 minutes.

Ceramic or stoneware pot
The longer you cook rice the easier it is to digest it. The flavour of rice changes when you use different types of equipment to cook it in. It seems a little sweeter in a ceramic or stoneware pot. Soak the rice 1 – 2 hours before cooking, using 1.5 – 2 parts water to 1 part rice. Place the pot over a medium heat and bring to the boil. Lower the heat, cover and simmer 40 – 45 minutes. Remove from heat and set aside for 10 minutes.

NOTE: If you soak the rice prior to cooking, always use the soaking water to cook the rice. Discarding this water means throwing away precious minerals.

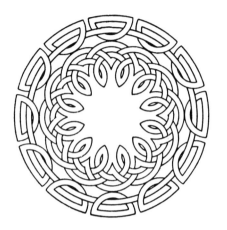

TOTAL APPROACH TO WELL-BEING

Eastern philosophy proposes that all forms of life in the universe are animated by an essential 'vital essence and vital force' called *'Ki'* (a Japanese word pronounced 'key' or *'Qi'* (a Chinese word pronounced 'chee'). These terms also translate as 'breath and air', and are similar to the Hindu concept of *prana*. *Ki* is a difficult concept to describe in words, especially in Northern European languages. The Greeks had a term 'quintessence', 'quint' meaning five and 'essence' translating as 'the body of a thing'. They also subscribed to a theory of what they called the four 'essences' of all creation: Fire, Earth, Air and Water, which are similar to the Chinese system of the Five Elements. However, underlying all these 'essences' was something called 'quintessence' which could not be accurately described in the Greek language.

THE CONCEPT OF *KI*

The Japanese term *Ki* is described as a quality that permeates all things throughout the universe (yet is not the same as the universe) and is close to the 'essence' of all things. When it comes to the human body, we talk about *Ki* in terms of human life force and essence. If there is a DEFICIENCY of *Ki*, it doesn't mean that there is no *Ki*; it means that there is a deficient QUANTITY of *Ki* in the body, or in other words, 'decreased life'. If a person dies, they still have *Ki*, but it is not referred to as human *Ki*.

In the human organism, aspects of *Ki* are often divided into the two qualities of Yin and Yang, the Yang being that which is vital and moving, and the Yin being nutritive. For example, blood is thought to be primarily Yin in quality as it moves slowly and nourishes the body. Yin *Ki* and blood are in fact often closely allied, the symptoms which arise from a deficiency of Yin being mainly connected with a deficiency of blood: a person feels 'false heat' with symptoms such as flushing, heat rising into the head, and thirstiness in the mouth without any real desire to drink. Conversely the symptoms that arise from a deficiency of Yang are coldness, weakness, the surface of the skin becoming easily chilled or sweating spontaneously, or a feeling of being run down with no energy.

When we talk about *Ki*, what we are talking about is the wholeness of human functioning, which can be differentiated into various categories such as nutritive energy, defensive energy (which acts like an envelope to protect us from things like wind or people who may have a negative effect) and spirit, in the sense of alertness, positiveness and aliveness.

All the organs and tissues of the body depend upon the flow of blood and *Ki* for normal and healthy functioning. Simultaneously, the activity and production of

MACROBIOTICS & BEYOND

blood and *Ki* depend upon the normal functioning of the viscera and bowels. Therefore, when a dis-ease state arises in a particular organ, it can affect the blood and *Ki* of that organ and may also affect the blood and *Ki* of the whole body as well.

Ki is transferable and transmutable: for example, digestion extracts *Ki* from food and drink and transfers it to the lungs. When air and essence of food meet, they transmute to form human *Ki*, which then circulates throughout the body as 'vital force and essence'. The quality and quantity and balance of your *Ki* determines your state of well-being and the span of your life. The key to maintaining optimum health is to establish a natural and harmonious balance among the vital energies within the body, as well as between those of the body and the external environment. The most important factors concerning *Ki*, however, are food, drink, stress, the air that we breathe, and how we breathe.

Character for *Ki* or *Qi* (both Japanese and Chinese): 气
The character is formed from these words:

Steam

Pot

Rice

Ki is like steam rising from cooking rice.

FOOD AND *KI*

Food can be termed 'warm' in terms of its energy-giving qualities, as well as being physically warm from cooking. The 'heat' in food is dependent upon its *Ki* vitality. Food that is stale, adulterated, processed or kept for too long as a leftover from a previous meal is without its essence. Although it is physically present, it lacks the 'fire of life' that supports the stomach *Ki*. Once food has been cooked it is best to eat it within twenty-four hours, and whenever there are leftovers, they should not be kept refrigerated too long, as re-heating destroys more of the 'vital essence' of the food. The purest essence of the food is in its smell, and the loss of aroma is an indication that the food is 'lifeless'.

In terms of this 'vital essence', food should ideally be organically grown, freshly picked or foraged, and as free as possible from toxins such as preservatives, insecticides, heavy metals and pollutants. However, certain cultured foods such as unpasteurised miso, yoghurt, and fermented pickles and sauerkraut should not be considered 'lifeless' as they are alive even though stored for long periods of time. (This is especially true if the foods concerned are not pasteurised.)

Autumn and winter are the times for storing and tonifying; spring and summer are the times for cleansing and eliminating. This is very important in terms of diet; if the seasons are not considered when choosing foods to eat, dis-ease can manifest the following season. In winter, for example, it is appropriate to eat foods that will move the energy of the body *down* to the core and regenerate essence and repair substance. In the warmer weather it is appropriate to eat foods which move the energy *up* to the surface, increasing elimination, such as those foods which induce perspiration and make the blood and *Ki* move quickly and freely.

In the northern hemisphere, seasonal diet is to a certain extent part of tradition; for example, Christmas dinner is well designed for the energetic needs of winter weather. It is a pity that in the southern hemisphere, where the climate is very different, people continue to celebrate traditional occasions such as Christmas with food that is most unsuitable for the time of year.

THE FIVE ELEMENTS, FLAVOURS AND ENERGIES

The theory of the Five Elements evolved from the Chinese philosophy of Taoism which divided the world into five symbolic elements: Wood, Fire, Earth, Metal and Water. Everything on Earth is seen to be dominated by one of these elements, and their constant interplay — combined with those of Yin and Yang — explain all change and activity in Nature.

The Chinese were an agrarian people who depended on their ability to live in harmony with Nature for survival. Through their experience they learned that just as there are five elements in the outside world, the same energies exist within each and everyone of us. The relationships among the elements are both generative and subjugative, and influence each other's force:

Generative cycle
Wood burns to generate Fire.
Fire produces ashes.
This generates Earth.
Earth generates Metal, which can be mined from the ground.
When heated Metal becomes molten, like Water.
Water promotes growth of plants, thereby generating Wood.

Subjugative cycle
Plants, represented by Wood, subjugate Earth by breaking up the soil and depleting its nutrients.
Earth subjugates Water by containing it in one place and soiling its clarity.
Water subjugates Fire by extinguishing it.
Fire subjugates Metal by melting it.
Metal subjugates Wood by cutting it.

Each vital organ belongs by nature to one of the Five Elements. Thus by understanding the relationships between the Five Elements you can understand how the vital organs interact and influence each other.

In disease conditions, the Chinese recognise an imbalance in one or more of the elements:

Symptom	**Imbalance**
Hot fever or excessive metabolic rate	FIRE
Chills or a low metabolic rate	WATER
Moving pain such as headache, common cold and arthritis	WIND
Dry diseases such as constipation, skin diseases and cough	METAL
Damp diseases such as weak digestion, edema and loose stools	EARTH

Generally, Hot and Dry arise together, Cold and Damp arise together, and WIND diseases can be either Hot or Cold.

Therapeutically, Chinese medicine is allopathic; it treats by opposite. However, subtle distinctions are important.

A seemingly Hot disease can arise from a deficiency of Yin — its opposite.

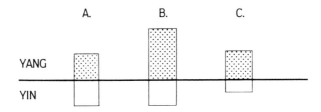

A. is a figurative balance of Yin/Yang.
B. is a true fever — an excess of Yang (Hot) energy.
C. is false fever, arising out of a deficiency of the Yin (Cooling) energy.

The Five Element theory is traditionally used to promote balance within the body organs, tissues, senses, secretions, and mental and spiritual states, as well as to promote balance in the way they react within the larger cosmos. Although a certain food or flavour may be supportive for an organ in small or moderate amounts, too much of the same food or flavour can deplete or harm the body.

It would be an error to be too simplistic and say for example that because the bitter flavour belongs to the Fire element, and summer is ruled by fire that bitter food should be eaten in the summer. There is no indication in the Chinese classics that bitter food is prescribed for the summer. Because of the linear way of thinking that inhabits the Western mind, we have tried to make rigid rules and charts that make us feel more secure.

W E L L — B E I N G

Yin and Yang and the Five Elements tie Chinese Medicine directly to traditional Chinese Philosophy and describe the human body in terms of the universal patterns of nature. There is no mention of eating flavours according to the seasons. The best way to use the Five Element theory is preventatively. What the Five Element Theory is showing us is what could happen if we overindulge.

Chinese philosophy describes food as falling into the categories of five basic flavours. The Five Flavours are sweet, sour, salty, bitter and pungent, and they each act in a different way on the internal organs of the human body. According to Henry C. Lu in *The Chinese System of Food Cures*, 'the common actions' of foods in terms of their flavours are as follows:

—Sweet foods (e.g. honey, tofu, kidney bean, wheat) can slow down acute symptoms and neutralise the toxic effects of other foods.

—Sour foods (e.g. plum and lemon) can obstruct internal movements, and are thus useful in checking diarrhoea and excessive perspiration.

—Salty foods (e.g. seaweed) can soften hardness, which explains their usefulness in treating painful obstructions and other symptoms involving the hardening of muscles or glands.

—Bitter foods (e.g. hops, daikon greens) can reduce body heat, dry body fluids, and induce bowel movement.

—Pungent foods (e.g. ginger, green onion and peppermint) can induce perspiration and promote energy circulation.

Food is also seen by the Chinese in terms of its ability to create different sensations within the body. The energies generated by foods are perceived as being of five types: hot, cold, warm, cool and neutral. Hot foods, for example, create warming sensations (through increasing metabolic function), while cold foods cool the body down (through decreasing metabolic function). However, the energy of a food refers only to its *effect* on the body. Even though you drink tea hot most of the time, it in fact has a cold energy; even if you eat chicken cold, you are still eating a warm food.

Energies and flavours of foods are also classified into Yin and Yang. Hot and warm energies are Yang; cool and cold energies are Yin. Pungent and sweet flavours are Yang; sour, bitter and salty flavours are Yin. When foods are classified into Yin and Yang both the energy and flavour of the food must be considered. Sometimes the energy of a food may be Yang and its flavour Yin, rather than saying that a food is either Yin or Yang. A better way of thinking about Yin and Yang is to say that one is MORE Yin or more Yang than another, thereby making things relative.

To put all of our eggs in one basket such as Yin/Yang would be quite foolish and even dangerous. Other phenomena should be taken into account, such as the five Natures, Taste, Yin/Yang and Four/Directions. Here are some simple explanation of these classifications so that you may begin to incorporate them into your lifestyle,

137

(see also History of Macrobiotics, page 15).

'Actions of Foods in the Seasonal Recipes' on page 168 lists the energetic actions created by the seasonal recipes at the front of this book. The chart on page 163 lists various foods and their associated organs, energies and flavours.

ASSESSING YOUR NEEDS

When designing a balanced diet for yourself or your family, it is wise to choose a mixture of different flavours and energies to suit individual needs and conditions. Here are some guidelines:

—If you have a hot physical constitution, choose more foods with a cold or cool energy; when choosing flavour, eat more bitter and only a very small amount of pungent foods.

—If you have a cold physical constitution, choose foods that are generally hot or warm in energy, and more sweet and pungent in flavour, using less bitter tasting foods.

— If you have a damp physical constitution, eat more foods that dry out the dampness and allow the water to pass out of the body more easily, avoiding foods that can produce fluids; use pungent and mildly sweet flavours.

—If you have a dry physical constitution, choose foods that can circulate energy and brown rice malt syrup or maltose and avoid foods that dry dampness like adzuki (red) beans and pumpkin.

—If you have an excessive constitution, choose foods that can circulate energy and blood; and avoid foods that will stagnate your energy.

—If you have a deficient constitution, choose more foods that can tonify such as red dates, chicken broth and yams. Avoid too many bitter-tasting foods.

These guidelines also apply to daily changes in one's condition. In this case, it is necessary to note the condition of the organs and the way in which they respond to daily lifestyle, activity, weather, food, etc. Each individual has different strengths and weaknesses, and these vary from day to day.

We should also remember other factors which contribute to health and longevity. Health and well-being are to a large extent in harmony with the larger flow of the universe — physically, mentally, emotionally and spiritually.

Other healing techniques, such as Chinese herbalism, acupuncture and shiatsu, are also based on the idea that the body is an energy field called *Ki* — an energy which is constantly being re-charged from the universe, entering the body and flowing along certain pathways called meridians. These techniques are a good support system to use in conjunction with a macrobiotic diet.

138

WELL — BEING

INDIVIDUALITY

Each person has a unique set of nutritional requirements for maintaining health and well-being. Some people, for example, require more of one food or less of another. Several factors influence what our needs are:
— activity level
— where we live
— the type of work that we do
— age
— sex
— degree of psychological and emotional stress
— genetics
— childhood eating patterns
— childhood stress patterns
— social habits (drinking, smoking)

We are all radically different in terms of these factors — and this is all part of our individuality. There are some people who eat salt excessively, but do not show signs of high blood pressure. Some smokers live to a ripe old age, whereas others do not. The real truth is that there is no one way, no one diet, and that 'One man's meat can be another man's poison'.

So just because your friend swears by a diet that works for him or her, it doesn't mean that it will necessarily work for you. Too many factors are involved in choosing foods that will nourish and support your well-being.

Life force or *Ki* is one of the most important considerations, and must be taken into account when considering what works and what doesn't. If a person constantly eats restaurant food and is not feeling healthy, it would be worthwhile to think about the *Ki* that might or might not be present in the food. After all, restaurant food does not have the same attention that home-cooking does, and is usually not prepared with the same amount of individual care and love. I sincerely believe that you receive the *Ki* of the person(s) responsible for the preparation and serving of the food you are eating.

One evening I had dinner at a macrobiotic food restaurant in New York City. I had often eaten at this particular restaurant, but that night after dinner I had a very strong sensation. The best way to describe it would be to say that I felt very peaceful, and well-loved. I enquired as to who the cook was on this particular evening and the owner said that a new person had been cooking for the past week. She described him as the most orderly, happy, sincere and loving person who had ever entered the kitchen, and she herself felt much more peaceful and calm after eating his food.

I would describe this incident as a strong example of the cook's *Ki* having entered the food. The message that this experience carried with it was a very powerful

139

one for me, one that made me reflect on my own organisation in the kitchen, and the way I felt when I was preparing food for myself and others. No matter what we ultimately choose to eat, the way it was grown, harvested, tended to, shipped, prepared, cooked, served and received will no doubt be reflected in the way that food nourishes us.

A LITTLE BIT OF WHAT YOU FANCY DOES YOU GOOD

Whether a food is good or bad for you depends upon the individual situation and even this can change from one moment to the next. Many foods have been labelled 'bad' by different alternative health groups without considering other necessary aspects of condition on a personal basis. For example, the statement that 'sugar is bad for everyone', should really be that '*too much* sugar is bad'.

It's also very popular to question the consumption of meat nowadays, and like sugar it too can have a place in the diets of some of us some of the time. Because we (as a race) have over-consumed many foods, meat being just one example, there is a current swing away from heavy meat-eating, with a trend towards lighter foods in general. (By the way, if you are thinking of decreasing your meat or sugar consumption, or abstaining from them completely, the transition from one food to another should be very gradual.)

Some people avoid certain foods altogether because they tend to be mucus-forming (for example, dairy products), but again let me stress that in small amounts these foods may be O.K. — unless your digestion is weak or you are 'sensitive' to them. Only you can know what works for you and it is just a case of trial and error until you learn what is suitable and what isn't. In addition, it's worth remembering that quality and gratitude plays a very large part in how our body responds to the foods which we put into it.

YIN AND YANG AND DIET

Yin-Yang theory is based on the philosophical construct of two polar complements, called *Yin* and *Yang*. [1] They are just labels used to describe how things function in relation to each other, and to a greater extent in the cosmos. They describe the process of change — continual change — and they are a way of thinking that is seen as part of a whole system, where all things in the universe are included. Nothing can exist in and of itself; nothing can be isolated from its relationship to other things and within each other, Yin and Yang always contain the possibility of change.

Yin and Yang, in our own bodies, are symbolised by Fire and Water, which represent the dynamic polarity that occurs within us. According to the Chinese system of classical medicine, all foods are not classified into *Yin* and *Yang* categories, but are made up of a complex of both *Yin* and *Yang* factors and can be *Yin* in terms of temperature or direction, and *Yang* in terms of flavour. The polarity of *Yin* and *Yang* is what is useful when we want to strike a balance between health and sickness, for example.

The original meaning of 'Yang', according to Ted Kaptchuk, in his book, *The Web That has no Weaver*, was the sunny side of a slope. The term implies brightness and is part of one common Chinese expression for the sun. *Yang* is associated with qualities such as heat, stimulation, movement, activity, excitement, vigor, light exteriority, upwardness, outwardness, and increase.

'The character for *Yin* originally meant the shady side of a slope. It is associated with such qualities as cold, rest, responsiveness, passivity, darkness, interiority, downwardness, inwardness and decrease.'

The time for cleansing and for nourishing too are based on the laws of *Yin* and *Yang* and act in relationship to the seasons. Spring and Summer are the times for cleansing, and Winter and Autumn the times for nourishing (tonifying and storing). Energy is naturally moving up and out in the Spring and Summer time so the body naturally opens up anyway to react with the environment to prevent illness by cleansing itself. In the Winter it is more appropriate to eat foods that move the energy down that will tonify the kidneys and the Middle Burner, (stomach/spleen) repair substance and regenerate Essence.

If we are truly interested in *Preventive* dietary therapy it is important to look at food from various perspectives. Quantity, whether we eat too little or too much, can create imbalance in our system. If one has little interest in food, one cannot produce

---

1. Kaptchuk, T. J., *The Web That has no Weaver*, Congdon & Weed, New York 1983. p. 8

MACROBIOTICS & BEYOND

sufficient Blood and *Ki* to nourish the function of the various organs. Conversely, if one overeats, the system becomes clogged and therefore the movement of Blood and *Ki* will be disturbed and this will eventually affect the function of the organs. This will eventually result in Deficiency, harming the digestive system and there also could be possible secondary problems in circulation. In either case, whether it be from overeating or undereating the result will be the same: Blood and *Ki* will stagnate which means that all life functioning eventually has no other choice but to cease.

Deficiency can also result when there is a lack of fire or warmth. These days, it is very popular to cleanse through colonics, fasts or choosing one 'eliminating' food such as raw vegetable juices and fruit juices to help move 'toxins' out of the body. However, from the Oriental perspective, toxemia is not the only cause of disease. According to Bob Flaws and Honora Wolfe in their book, *Prince Wen Hui's Cook, Chinese Dietary Therapy*, Disease and ill health are caused by hypofunctioning of the internal organism, hyperfunctioning of the internal organs due to attenuation of the physical substrate, and invasion of the organism by External pathogenic factors due to poor resistance. Each of these three etiologies may be caused by lack of nutritious, tonifying foods which are usually considered warming, such as cooked vegetables, grains and small amounts of animal foods.

We must also consider the temperature of the food that we eat, both energetically and physically. Food that is too hot will damage the digestive organs, such as the stomach and intestines. Conversely, food that is too cold will put out the Middle Burner Fire (stomach/spleen). Energetically, the heat of a food is dependent upon its *Ki* or vitality. When food is old, processed or highly refined there is no *Ki* left in it.

So Oriental diets stress mainly cooked foods to maintain the life-force of the Middle Burner. The belief that cooked foods should predominate in a person's diet stems from the desire not to harm the digestive Fire. Foods must be chewed well, and eaten in moderation. Not too much liquid should be consumed as it can smother the Fire and cause Water toxin. Even in the hot weather it is best not to eat too much frozen or iced foods as they do not support the Middle Burner. Best, of course, is the road of moderation to support preventive dietary therapy.

The definition of *Yin* and *Yang* from the classical Chinese medicine perspective is different than that used in the Macrobiotic sense. According to Chinese traditional medicine, *Yang* is active, aggressive, expansive, centrifugal, and negative. *Yin*, on the other hand, is contractive, internalising, centripetal, conservative and positive. All mention and use of the concepts of *Yin* and *Yang* in this book are made from the Chinese traditional point of view, as supported by the classical Chinese texts.

142

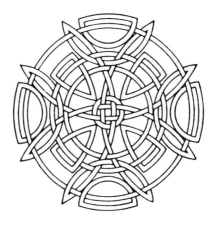

KITCHEN-WISE

MEAL PLANNING

When I began to give my son solid foods I found myself even more dedicated to using whole foods and also pressed for time. How did I do it? The key is top organisational techniques. For example, you will probably have leftovers such as grains and beans. (Most of the recipes in this book list ingredients in quantities which allow for leftovers.) Just add fresh vegetables, tofu, toasted seeds or nuts (which have already been toasted in the morning while preparing breakfast): you can stir fry the vegetables with leftover rice, blend leftover beans with tofu, tahini (or other nut butters), herbs, spices and fresh parsley, and bake all of this into a loaf. (Add a few eggs if you want to feed more than a few.) Add a side salad, and away you go.

After dinner, you can soak another quantity of grains or beans, toast some more nuts and seeds, or make a dip from leftover beans or tofu. If you know that you will be out for a few hours the following day, try toasting some grain, adding boiling water and some whole root vegetables, and baking it covered for several hours. (This is best in the colder months.) When you come home, dinner will be almost ready. Make sure that you set your oven very low to compensate for the long cooking time.

At the end of the week, before I shop for the following week's organic vegetables and fruits, I take out all the remaining leftover vegetables, slice them in various ways and toss them with leftover brown rice and barley flour. Then I add just enough water or stock until the mixture sticks together (when half a handful is squeezed in the hand). Test a half-handful by deep-frying it, and if the mixture sticks together you have put in the right amount of flour. (Avoid using watery vegetables such as lettuce or cucumbers as they make the mix too runny.) This may sound vague, but it is often the favourite meal of the week. Sometimes I add curry powder or cumin, or mix in a few dry herbs for a variation in flavour.

Try stuffing cooked or raw vegetables, such as zucchini, pumpkin or capsicum, with leftovers. The golden rule in my kitchen is, 'When food that has been a liquid is leftover, turn it into a solid, and when it has been solid create something liquid from it'. Soups turn into the most delicious loaves, pâtés or molds, and pies turn into scrumptious soups, sauces or thick gravies.

For dessert, I always have some extra crumb topping on hand (leftover from another dessert). Take some fresh fruit and cook it in a little fruit juice. Then dissolve 2 – 3 t kuzu or arrowroot flour in ½ cup cold juice or water and stir it into the fruit mixture. Add a little grated lemon rind if appropriate, or try five spice powder for a change of taste. Top with some crumb topping and watch it dissappear!

CONSIDERING TASTE, TEXTURE AND COLOUR

I often speak about balance and harmony, and this is also very important when considering the subtle blend of the five tastes: sour, sweet, salty, bitter and pungent (spicy). If these tastes are always included in each meal then the food will be satisfying to those who eat it. Place condiments on the table that also represent some or all of the five flavours so that those people who need more of one than another can help themselves.

We all like different textures in our foods throughout the day, and this is easily seen in the types of foods people like to indulge in — from the often-consumed packet of crunch chips to creamy desserts. You can create these textures in your own home-cooked meals by deep frying, blending beans, tofu and other ingredients together to make creamy dips, spreads and sauces, baking desserts that are both creamy and crunchy, and using raw carrots and celery for that added crunch.

Nature has provided us with a colourful selection of foods, and by using a variety of colours you can present very appealing and appetising meals. Toss grains with minced parsley and grated carrot, or pickles, place this in a mold and turn it upside down on lettuce leaves to serve. Use garnishes on soups that complement the colour of the soup. We really do eat with our eyes, and the best way to get people to try our cooking is to present food that says 'EAT ME'!

STORING FOODS

Most food items can be easily stored in glass, wooden, metal or ceramic containers. They should have tight-fitting lids to keep out insects and dust.

Flours, Beans, Seeds, Grains (uncooked)

If you live in a warm or hot climate, I suggest that you keep all of these foods refrigerated. It is also a good idea to put bay leaves in the food containers to discourage insects from sharing the premises. The most important points for grain storage are:
— cool temperature
— no light
— low humidity
— keep whole grains rather than cracked

The bran kernel was designed to preserve the grain. Wheatgerm and flours are the most susceptible to air and heat exposure as the oils are no longer sealed in. These in particular need refrigeration in the hot weather.

Fruits and Vegetables

Most vegetables and fruits, especially if they are organically and/or biodynamically grown, need a cool environment. Onions and some squash and pumpkin can keep in a basket, but make sure that the squash and pumpkin are not touching each other. Wrap greens in newspaper and refrigerate for best results. I find it best to remove all plastic bags from vegetables, especially greens and root vegetables, as they mould when moisture collects in the bag.

Tofu
Remove the tofu from its original container and place in a metal or ceramic bowl. Cover completely with cold water and change the water every other day. If the tofu smells 'sour', discard it.

Oils and Nut Butters
Refrigerate oils and nut butters (tahini, almond butter, etc.) and use as rapidly as possible. If you buy oil in bulk, change the container as the quantity changes. This procedure prevents an excessive amount of oxygen from accumulating in the container and mixing with the oil. It is best to use sesame oil as it contains a natural anti-rancidity agent called 'sesamol'.

Tamari, Shoyu and Miso
Keep these items in a cool, dry place. If you buy unpasteurised miso, keep it in a glass, ceramic or porcelain container in the refrigerator. Store tamari or shoyu in a dark glass container as light decomposes it.

Pickles
Keep pickles in a cool, dry place.

Sea Vegetables, Teas, Herbs and Spices
Keep these items covered, away from light and in a cool, dry place.

Leftovers
Look for containers that are made from glass, stainless steel, or ceramic and for a time saver tip, try corningware which can go straight from the refrigerator onto the stove or in the oven.

COOKWARE AND UTENSILS
If you are considering a change in your dietary habits, don't feel that you have to get rid of everything in the kitchen and buy a whole new set of cookware and utensils. Take stock of what you have and consider the *quality* of each item, and perhaps you

may want to add a thing or two. Here are some tips to keep in mind when purchasing new cookware:

— Make sure that saucepans are light enough for you to handle comfortably but heavy enough to conduct heat evenly. Lightweight saucepans tend to warp easily, especially when they do not have a thick copper base (if they are stainless steel). Saucepans that are too heavy cannot be handled properly.
— It is easier to work with saucepans that have sloping sides instead of perpendicular ones, so that stirring does not become awkward.
— Covers should fit tightly, with no gaps for steam to escape.
— Make sure that the cookware you choose is the most suitable type for your purposes. Stainless steel, cast iron, glass, porcelain or earthenware are most suitable for everyday use. I do not recommend Aluminum, teflon or any other nonstick coated cookware. Aluminum is absorbed into the food, while nonstick or plastic coatings are easily chipped, and the pieces can get mixed into the food.

Glass cookware does not leach anything into the food you are cooking. It does not peel or chip, and if food sticks to the pan it is easily removable. If you have any reaction to metal cookware then glass would be a good, safe alternative for you. However, glass is a poor conductor of heat; it heats slowly and does not distribute heat evenly. It would be wise to place a simmer ring underneath glass cookware after it has come to the boil. Always begin cooking with low heat. When cleaning glass, be sure to handle it carefully as harsh abrasives will scratch the surfaces.

I recommend using wooden utensils, which are durable and less likely to impart any taste into the food. wooden utensils can include soup ladles, bamboo rice paddles, spoons for stirring and mixing, and tongs for lifting. Here is some information on other kitchen utensils which you may find useful.

Cutting Boards
Wooden cutting boards are the best surfaces for doing any kind of cutting work. Whether it be vegetables, spices such as garlic or ginger, or fish, wood is the best surface to use. When you cut something like garlic or ginger or fish that has a strong odour, just rub salt into the board and rinse in cold water. Dry the board and give it a light coating of oil; this will help keep the surface smooth and workable. I suggest that you keep two or even three cutting boards: one for spices, one for vegetables and one for fish and chicken.

Vegetable Brushes
In order to clean your vegetables properly (especially root vegetables), try using vegetable scrubbing brushes. This will allow you to clean the vegetables without peeling them, thus retaining essential vitamins and minerals in the skin.

Heat Spreader (Disperser)

This is a round piece of metal which can be placed directly on the heat (gas or electric) to prevent food from burning.

Graters

There are many different kinds of graters available. I use a stainless steel grater for lemon rinds or grating carrots, etc., but when it comes to grating ginger, garlic or daikon (Japanese radish) a porcelain one is what I use — it does not alter the taste of strong spices such as ginger.

Suribachi

This Japanese mortar and pestle has always been a conversation piece in my cooking classes as well as at dinner parties. It can be used to make condiments, sauces, dressings, dips and even for puréeing baby foods. It's my favourite toy!

Appliances

Whenever possible I prefer to do most of my kitchen work with my own hands. Occasionally I use an electric processor for mixing or whipping cake batters, but when it comes to cutting I use a knife and a board.

BASIC CUTTING TECHNIQUES

All knives consist of three distinct parts: the tip, middle and base of the blade. Different parts of the knife are used to make different cuts.

Peeling

When peeling vegetables turn the knife on its side and use the base. Hold the vegetable firmly in one hand and place the knife along the surface of the vegetable and your thumb over the peel so that you assess the thickness and the depth of the cut. Place your index finger on top of the back of the blade to help the knife along.

Chopping, Mincing and Dicing

Chop the vegetables neatly and evenly. Then for mincing or dicing, hold the tip of the knife down on the cutting board with one hand and while working the rest of the blade up and down. Rotate it to the left and to the right so that you get an even chop.

Draw Cutting

Using only the tip of the knife, and holding the base well above the cutting board, draw the knife towards you in long even strokes, for thin or thick strips.

Push Cutting
Dense vegetables like onions, cabbage, turnips or swedes need to come in contact with the middle of the blade of the knife. As you cut, push slightly away and down, then up again and down, so that you actually create a circle.

Care and Cleaning of Knives
I like to use stainless steel or carbon steel vegetable knives for most of my cutting. After each use of the knife, wash it well in cold water only. If you have a carbon steel knife you may want to polish it as follows: Sprinkle some cleanser on the flat end of a piece of carrot or cabbage stem, and use it to polish both sides of the blade. Wash and rise thoroughly and wipe dry immediately. Alternatively, use a good quality stone to sharpen carbon steel knives.

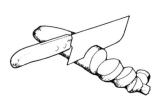

Rounds
This technique is simply cutting straight across the vegetable as thick or as thin as necessary. (The thicker the cut, the longer the cooking.)

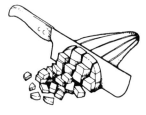

Dicing or mincing
For round vegetables, especially onions first cut the vegetable in half lengthwise. Then cutting towards the root thinly slice leaving the root intact. Then go the opposite way lengthwise as thick or as thin as you like. Finally chop across.

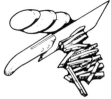

Matchsticks or Julienne
Cut the vegetables first on the diagonal, then pile them up *almost* on each other (like a fan effect) and cut lengthwise into thin strips.

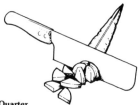

Quarter
Cut the vegetable in half lengthwise, then in half again lengthwise. Then cut across.

WATER AND FIRE

Cooking would be virtually impossible without water and fire. Filtered, spring, or well water which has not been chlorinated, fluoridated or treated with various other chemicals is naturally the best to use. If these choices are unavailable to you, always use boiled water for cooking or drinking.

K I T C H E N   W I S E

Most of us are beginning to recognise the need to pay close attention to the quality of our daily food, but in addition we now need to consider the quality of our daily 'fire', which cooks our food. Can the heat we choose to cook our daily foods affect our health and vitality?

Of the three most common cooking fuels — gas, electricity, and microwave radiation — it is the latter which tends to be questioned the most. The microwave is a form of radiant energy that occupies a central region of the electromagnetic spectrum of waves, which are very high frequency and vibrate at rates of millions to billions of cycles per second. Essentially, the microwave facilitates the food to cook itself, by making its own molecules vibrate so fast their motion produces the cooking fuel. Gas and electric stoves indirectly generate heat and transfer it from the burner to the food through the cookware, whereas microwaves cook by generating and transferring microwave energy *directly* to the foods without the intermediary of the cookware (according to Richard Leviton in *East West Journal*, June 1987, page 53).

There are many pros and cons for the microwave, and of course the biggest plus is the time-saving factor. However, even though studies have proven that microwave cooking retains a relatively high proportion of fragile nutrients compared with other methods, overcooking is a big problem because foods continue to cook even after they have been removed from the oven.

Basically the choice is up to us. Wood of course gives us the best flavour, and the most steady source of heat. However, it is not always practical. Gas is the next best fuel source, and electric would be my next choice.

As far as microwave ovens are concerned, it seems to me that when foods are cooked in a microwave oven they use their own energy to break themselves down, thereby getting less energy than what you started with.

Safety wise, it seems that numerous by-products are also released in the gas combustion process including sulphur dioxide, hydrogen cyanide, nitric oxide formaldehyde and vapours from organic chemicals. These can produce medical symptoms in a small number of extra sensitive people.

Microwave ovens also produce side effects, according to Dr Robert O. Becker, author of *The Body Electric* (William Morrow, 1985). Dr Becker suggests that even very low levels of exposure to microwave radiation, such as one might get from the use of the microwave in the home, can have serious health effects.

Personally, I would rather use a fuel that takes a little longer. The food from microwave ovens seems dead, lacking vitality or 'life force'. It's something that cannot be measured, but nevertheless the difference is there. When you spend extra time preparing food, when you work together creating harmony and balance, the food is a gift of love to yourself and to others; this in turn creates more 'life force' and vital energy (*Ki*).

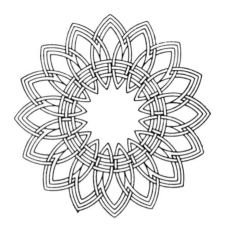

CHINESE SYSTEM OF DIAGNOSIS AND TREATMENT

COLD

SYMPTOM	SIGNS	METHOD OF TREATMENT	FOODS
EXTERNAL COLD			PUNGENT
Quick onset, brought about by chills and consuming cold food and drink.	Aversion to cold, cold limbs, dull stagnant look, white complexion, thin watery faeces, clear runny nose, pain in body and joints, watery vomit.	To cause perspiration and warm body.	anise, sweet basil, bay leaf, butter, camphor mint, capers, caraway seed, cardamon seed, cassia bark, chive, coriander, dill seed, fennel, garlic, ginger, greek onion, jasmine flower, leek, lemon peel, cumquat, tangerine peel, rosemary, safflower, shallot, spearmint, coriander, majoram, white pepper.
INTERNAL COLD			
Generally long term. A weakening of the body's *Yang Ki*.	Dislike of cold, cold limbs, vomiting of clear water, watery stool, edema, frequent urination, underactivity, sluggishness, abdominal swelling.	To warm and tone.	abalone, almonds, anchovy, apple, barley, lamb's brain, caraway seed, beef, dates, lotus seed, pork pancreas, cassia bark, dill seed, garlic, kidney bean, string bean, mung bean, beet, butterfish, capers, cardamon, cheese, cherry, chestnut, chicken, chive, coconut, corn, coriander, cucumber,

153

MACROBIOTICS & BEYOND

SYMPTOM	SIGNS	METHOD OF TREATMENT	FOODS
			egg, fennel, goose meat, honey, lamb/pork heart, mango, mutton, clove oil.

HEAT

SYMPTOM	SIGNS	METHOD OF TREATMENT	FOODS
TRUE HEAT	Fear of heat, high fever, restlessness, infrequent urination of dark colour, red tongue and complexion, agitation, diarrhoea.	To clear heat by sweating.	COLD AND PUNGENT FOODS apple, cucumber, mung bean, daikon, coconut, milk, bitter gourd, ice, lemon, ling, coconut oil, pineapple, watermelon pulp, lotus leaf and root, white pepper, wheatgerm, mandarin peel, clam, crab, preserved egg, kelp, nori, rabbit liver, octopus, salt, soy sauce, tomato.
FALSE HEAT Arises with deficiency of *Yin Ki* and there are usually no pathogens or infection.	Periodic fever, night sweats, feeling miserable, skinniness, dry mouth and throat. Usually a feeling of heat in the upper body and head and coldness and emptiness in the lower body.	To tonify *Yin*.	AVOID TOO MUCH COLD FOOD cheese, chicken/duck egg, pear peel, asparagus, abalone, kidney bean, castor bean, string bean, azuki bean, sword bean, beef, duck, millet, octopus, oyster, pork, sardine, shark meat, prawn.

CHINESE DIAGNOSIS AND TREATMENT

True heat can be EXTERNAL: Symptoms are those of sunstroke.

INTERNAL: Specific symptoms — Lung Heat: Yellow phlegm
Heat in Blood: Menstrual haemorrhage
Skin Heat: Skin eruption or itch.

Note: Any infection is usually considered a heat sign.

WIND

EXTERNAL WIND: Usually quick in onset, with symptom patterns changing rapidly.

SYMPTOM	SIGNS	METHOD OF TREATMENT	FOODS
WIND HEAT			COOLING AND PUNGENT FOODS
	Headache, red eyes, mental unclarity, blocked nose, cough, thirst, yellow sticky phlegm, red tongue, fear of wind, moving pain in body.	To clear heat, stop wind.	agar, sweet basil, peppermint, spearmint, peppermint oil, camphor mint, white pepper, wheatgerm, mandarine peel, asparagus, banana, crab, chinese endive, kelp, octopus, rice washing water, chinese long-leaved spinach, papaya.
WIND COLD			WARM AND PUNGENT FOODS
	Headache, mental unclarity, red eyes, blocked nose, cough, sore throat, generalised ache, thin clear phlegm, no thirst, fear of wind.	To disperse wind and cold.	anise, sweet basil, bay leaf, camphor mint, capers, caraway seed, cardamon seed, chive, coriander, dill seed, fennel, garlic, ginger, onion, onion juice, leek, lemon peel, cumquat, tangerine peel, rosemary, safflower, spring onion, spearmint, angelica

155

MACROBIOTICS & BEYOND

INTERNAL WIND			
More serious condition arising from long term imbalances.	Tremor, high fever, dizziness, paralysis, unclear consciousness.	To stop wind, nourish Blood and *Yin*, clear heat.	mulberry, cheese, pine nut kernel, cuttlefish, chicken egg/membrane, beef liver, pork liver, nutmeg, oyster (fresh), sea cucumber, spinach.

DAMP

SYMPTOM	SIGNS	METHOD OF TREATMENT	FOODS
EXTERNAL DAMP			
Transitory and arises with the weather	Swelling and heavy sensations of head and body with fatigue, congested chest, sticky sensation in mouth.	To cause mild perspiration and remove dampness.	alfalfa root, azuki bean, capers, lotus flowers, coriander, ginger, green onion, marjoram, white pepper, rosemary.
INTERNAL DAMP			
Results from long duration of worry, poor food and excess of food and drink	Poor appetite, abdominal swelling, heaviness and fatigue, loose stools but not necessarily diarrhoea.	To dry dampness with bitter flavour and warm energy.	tangerine peel, pine leaf, azuki bean, butterfish, celery, crab-apple, endive, flour, hops, kohlrabi, lettuce, liver of lamb, rabbit and pork, loquat, papaya, peach, pumpkin, radish leaf, rye, sago, turnip, vinegar, asparagus, ginseng.

Note: Damp is heavy and difficult to change. It is stagnation.

CHINESE DIAGNOSIS AND TREATMENT

FOODS TO BE AVOIDED IN DAMP CONDITIONS:
milk and milk products, pork, shark meat, egg, sardine, agar, asparagus, bamboo shoot, black sesame, cabbage, clam, mussel, crab, octopus, coconut milk, cucumber, duck, goose, seaweed, kelp, kudzu, olive, soybean, tofu, spinach, pinenut

FOODS TO BE AVOIDED IN WIND CONDITIONS:
eggs, all fats of any description, shrimp, prawns, sugar

DRY

SYMPTOM	SIGNS	METHOD OF TREATMENT	FOODS
EXTERNAL			
	Usually respiratory — dry cough, dry throat and lungs, dry lips and nostrils, rough chapped skin, little sputum, possible nosebleeds.	Stimulate Lung *Ki*.	agar, asparagus, soybean drink, duck egg, olive, bean curd, chicken egg, honey, sesame oil, pear, pork, spinach, leaf mustard, almond, apricot seed, crab apple, lemon juice, loquat, thyme.
INTERNAL			SWEET FLAVOUR AND COLD ENERGY
A long term condition arising from damage to *Yin Ki*.	Dry skin and hair, withered fingernails, dry and cracked lips, dry cough, thirst, feeling hunger frequently, dry stools.	To water *Yin* lubricate dryness to produce fluids.	cheese, asparagus, soybean drink, duck/chicken egg, olive, bean curd, honey, sesame oil, peach kernel, pear, pork, sea cucumber, soybean, angelica.

Note: Dry will arise with heat diseases, so treat heat sign first and see if dryness subsides.

BLOOD DEFICIENCY

SYMPTOM	SIGNS	METHOD OF TREATMENT	FOODS
BLOOD DEFICIENCY	Withered yellow complexion, numbness or weak tremors in limbs, emaciation, dizziness, poor sleep with night sweating, palpitations, poor shen (no inspiration).	To tonify Blood/*Yin*.	abalone, agar, anchovy, anise, apple, asparagus, bamboo shoot, banana, barley, kidney bean, castor bean, mung, beet, butter, butterfish, caraway seed, celery, cheese, cherry, chestnut, chicken, coconut, corn, cucumber, date, duck, eel, chicken/duck egg, fig, gluten, goose, grape, honey, lamb kidney, lettuce, chicken/beef/lamb/rabbit liver, loquat, mackerel, mango, marjoram, millet, shiitake mushroom, mutton, octopus, oyster, papaya, peach, pear, pineapple, pork, sweet potato, potato, pumpkin, rabbit, radish, sweet rice, shark, shrimp, spinach.

Note: Cold foods should be avoided in deficiency conditions.

CHINESE DIAGNOSIS AND TREATMENT

KI DEFICIENCY

SYMPTOM	SIGNS	METHOD OF TREATMENT	FOODS
KI DEFICIENCY	General fatigue, lack of strength, lack of physical vitality, short shallow breathing, no energy to speak, faint low voice, short of breath with simplest movement.	Tonify *Ki/ Yang.*	lamb's brain, rice bran, butter, butterfish, camphor mint, capers, caraway, cardamon, cherry, chestnut, chicken, red chili, chive, chrysthemum leaf, coconut milk, coriander, date, dill seed, eel, fennel, garlic, ginger, onion, guava, lamb kidney, kohlrabi, leek, lemon peel, marjoram, chicken/pork liver, mussel, beef/lamb marrow, mutton, nutmeg, soybean oil, peach, pearl sago, radish, sweet potato, rosemary, shrimp, squash, trout, turnip, vinegar, ginseng, prawn.

COLD FOODS

agar, alfalfa/mung sprouts, asparagus, bamboo shoot, banana, water chestnut, clam, crab, endive, grapefruit, kelp, nori, rabbit liver, mulberry, octopus, peppermint, rice water, salt, soy paste, wheatgerm, bitter endive, mandarin peel.

WARM FOODS

anchovy, anise, sweet basil, bay leaf, lamb's brain, butterfish, capers, caraway, cardamon, cherry, chestnut, chicken, chive, coconut, coriander, dates, dill seed, eel, fennel, garlic, green onion, mussel, leek, lamb kidney, mutton, nutmeg, peach, pine nut, sweet potato, rosemary, squash, vinegar, ginseng, prawn.

THE FIVE FOOD FLAVOURS

SWEET
abalone, agar, almond, anchovy, anise, apple, asparagus, bamboo shoot, banana, barley, string bean, azuki bean, mung bean, bean curd, beet, butterfish, cabbage, caraway, carrot, celery, cherry, chestnut, chicken, coconut, corn, cucumber, date, eel, egg, endive, fig, grape, lamb kidney, nori, shiitake, chicken/lamb/beef liver, mutton, peas, peach, plum, potato, shrimp, turnip.

PUNGENT
anise, bay leaf, sweet basil, capers, red chili, cardamon, chive, coriander, dill, fennel, garlic, ginger, onion, kohlrabi, leek, lemon peel, nutmeg, cumquat, radish, rosemary, spearmint, taro, watercress, wheatgerm, wild celery.

BITTER
alfalfa, red bean, asparagus, capers, butterfish, celery, crab-apple, endive, flour, hops, kohlrabi, lettuce, lamb/rabbit/pork liver, loquat, papaya, turnip, vinegar, ginseng.

SOUR
azuki bean, cheese, crab shell, grape, grapefruit, lemon peel, mango, olive oil, peach, plum, pomegranate, raspberry, tomato, strawberry, trout, vinegar, mandarin, coriander seed.

SALTY
abalone, barley, clam, crab, dill seed, duck, kelp, pork kidney, nori, rabbit liver, mussel, octopus, oyster, pork, salt, sardine, prawn.

MOVEMENT OF FOODS

DIRECTION	FOODS	SYMPTOMS	FLAVOURS	SEASONS
Upward (from lower region to upper)	(greens, sprouting, above ground vegetables) asparagus, beef, beetroot, black fungus (chinese), black sesame seeds, chinese cabbage, carrot, cherry	diarrhoea	warm and hot pungent and sweet flavour	Spring
Downward (upper to lower region)	(fruits, seeds and roots) apple, banana, barley, bean curd, chicken, egg white, button mushroom, cucumber, eggplant, lettuce, litchi, mango, mung bean, peach, persimmon, spinach, strawberry, tangerine, watermelon, wheat, wheat bran	vomiting, asthma, hiccupping	cold or cool or warm foods. Sweet or sour foods.	Autumn
Outward (inside to outside)	(spices, flowers, leaves) black pepper, cinnamon bark, dried ginger, green and red pepper, soybean oil, white pepper, peppermint	induce perspiration and reduce fever	hot energy, pungent or sweet foods	Summer

Inward (outside to inside)	(grains, seeds and nuts) banana, clams (salt and freshwater) crab, hops, kelp, lettuce, salt, seaweed, sour foods	ease bowel movements and abdominal swelling	cold energy, bitter or salty	Winter
Glossy (sliding)	honey, spinach	constipation and internal dryness		
Obstructive	guava, olive	diarrhoea and seminal emission, excessive perspiration, frequent urination		

Foods prepared with wine have a tendency to move upwards.
Foods prepared with ginger juice have a tendency to move outwards.
Foods prepared with vinegar have a tendency to be obstructive.
Foods prepared with salt have a tendency to move downwards (usually fried and salted foods).

FOODS AND THEIR ASSOCIATED ORGANS, ENERGIES AND FLAVOURS

	LUNGS	LGE. INTESTINE	STOMACH	SPLEEN	HEART	SM. INTESTINE	BLADDER	KIDNEY	PERICARDIUM	TRIP. HEATER	GALL BLADDER	LIVER	COLD	HOT	COOL	WARM	NEUTRAL	SLIDING	PUNGENT	SWEET	TASTELESS	SOUR	HARSH	BITTER	SALTY
Aduki Beans					✓	✓											✓			✓	✓				
Agar-Agar	✓										✓	✓						✓		✓					
Alfalfa																	✓							✓	
Almond	✓																✓		✓						
Almond Butter																	✓		✓						
Apple															✓					✓					
Apple Juice															✓					✓					
Apricot	✓	✓															✓			✓					
Arame													✓												✓
Asparagus															✓									✓	
Bamboo Shoot													✓							✓					
Banana													✓							✓					
Barley Flour															✓										✓
Basil	✓	✓		✓		✓										✓			✓						
Bay Leaf																✓			✓						
Beetroot																✓				✓					
Bifun Noodle																✓				✓					
Black Bean																✓				✓					
Blackberries																				✓		✓			
Black Pepper							✓												✓						
Black Olive	✓	✓														✓				✓		✓	✓		
Black Sesame Seed					✓			✓								✓				✓					
Blueberries																				✓		✓			
Brandy																✓			✓					✓	
Bread													✓							✓				✓	
Breadcrumbs													✓							✓				✓	
Broad Bean			✓	✓													✓			✓					
Brown Rice			✓	✓													✓			✓					
Brown Rice Flour																	✓			✓					

MERIDIANS ROUTES   ENERGIES   FLAVOURS

MACROBIOTICS & BEYOND

	Lungs	Lge. Intestine	Stomach	Spleen	Heart	Sm. Intestine	Bladder	Kidney	Pericardium	Trip. Heater	Gall Bladder	Liver	Cold	Hot	Cool	Warm	Neutral	Sliding	Pungent	Sweet	Tasteless	Sour	Harsh	Bitter	Salty
Brown Rice Malt	✓		✓	✓												✓				✓					
Brown Rice Vinegar			✓									✓				✓						✓		✓	
Buckwheat		✓	✓	✓											✓					✓					
Bulghur Wheat																				✓		✓		✓	
Butternut Pumpkin																	✓			✓				✓	
Button Mushroom	✓	✓	✓	✓				✓												✓					
Capsicum																✓									
Capers																✓			✓					✓	
Caraway			✓			✓										✓			✓	✓					
Cardamon	✓			✓												✓			✓						
Carrot	✓			✓													✓			✓					
Cashew Nut Butter																✓				✓					
Celery			✓									✓			✓					✓				✓	
Cherry																✓				✓		✓			
Chestnut			✓	✓			✓									✓				✓					
Chicken			✓	✓												✓				✓					
Chili				✓	✓									✓					✓						
Chives																✓			✓						
Cinnamon																			✓						
Cloves															✓				✓						
Coconut																	✓			✓					
Cognac																✓			✓	✓				✓	
Coriander Leaves	✓			✓												✓			✓						
Coriander Seed																✓			✓			✓			
Corn																	✓			✓					
Cucumber		✓	✓	✓				✓							✓					✓					
Currants																				✓					
Dates			✓	✓												✓				✓					
Dill																✓			✓	✓					
Dill Seed			✓			✓										✓			✓						
Egg																	✓			✓					
Eggwhite															✓					✓					
Eggyolk				✓		✓											✓			✓					
Eggplant		✓	✓	✓											✓					✓				✓	
Endive													✓											✓	
Endive (Bitter)		✓	✓	✓	✓								✓											✓	

MERIDIANS ROUTES   ENERGIES   FLAVOURS

FOODS, ENERGIES AND FLAVOURS

	LUNGS	LGE. INTESTINE	STOMACH	SPLEEN	HEART	SM. INTESTINE	BLADDER	KIDNEY	PERICARDIUM	TRIP. HEATER	GALL BLADDER	LIVER	COLD	HOT	COOL	WARM	NEUTRAL	SLIDING	PUNGENT	SWEET	TASTELESS	SOUR	HARSH	BITTER	SALTY
English spinach		✓				✓										✓				✓					
Fennel																✓			✓	✓					
Fig	✓	✓		✓													✓			✓					
Five Spice Powder																✓			✓						
Flour — Whole Wheat												✓								✓				✓	
Fruit Juice																				✓					
Garlic	✓		✓	✓												✓			✓						
Ginger	✓		✓	✓												✓			✓						
Ginger Juice																✓			✓						
Golden Squash			✓	✓								✓								✓					
Green Beans				✓				✓									✓			✓					
Green Chili				✓	✓							✓							✓						
Hazelnut																✓				✓					
Kidney Bean																	✓			✓	✓				
Kombu			✓	✓									✓							✓					✓
Kudzu			✓										✓							✓					
Leek																✓			✓				✓		
Lemon																						✓			
Lemon Pepper																			✓	✓					
Lemon Rind																✓			✓			✓			
Lettuce	✓	✓										✓												✓	
Lime																			✓		✓				
Lotus Leaf			✓	✓								✓				✓							✓	✓	
Lotus Seed (Fresh)			✓	✓		✓										✓				✓		✓			
Lotus Seed (Dried)			✓	✓		✓										✓				✓		✓			
Maltose	✓		✓	✓												✓				✓					
Mandarin															✓					✓		✓			
Mango															✓					✓		✓			
Maple Syrup																				✓					
Marsala																	✓				✓				
Millet			✓	✓		✓									✓					✓					✓
Mochi	✓		✓	✓												✓				✓					
Mung Sprout													✓							✓					
Mushroom (Cloud Ear)		✓											✓		✓					✓					
Mushroom (Button)	✓	✓	✓	✓											✓					✓					
Mushroom (Shiitake)			✓														✓			✓					

MERIDIANS ROUTES   ENERGIES   FLAVOURS

165

MACROBIOTICS & BEYOND

	LUNGS	LGE. INTESTINE	STOMACH	SPLEEN	HEART	SM. INTESTINE	BLADDER	KIDNEY	PERICARDIUM	TRIP. HEATER	GALL BLADDER	LIVER	COLD	HOT	COOL	WARM	NEUTRAL	SLIDING	PUNGENT	SWEET	TASTELESS	SOUR	HARSH	BITTER	SALTY
Mustard	✓																								
Mustard Seed	✓																								
Nori													✓							✓					✓
Nutmeg		✓		✓												✓			✓						
Oats																✓	✓			✓					
Olive	✓		✓													✓				✓		✓	✓		
Onion																✓			✓						
Orange Rind	✓			✓												✓			✓	✓					
Peach																✓				✓		✓			
Peanut Butter	✓			✓													✓			✓					
Pear	✓		✓									✓								✓					
Pepper (Black)														✓					✓						
Pine Nut	✓	✓						✓								✓				✓					
Potato																	✓			✓					
Prawns	✓			✓	✓		✓	✓				✓				✓				✓					✓
Pumpkin																	✓			✓				✓	
Radish	✓		✓												✓				✓	✓					
Raspberry																	✓			✓		✓			
Rice			✓	✓													✓			✓					
Rice Flour																	✓			✓					
Rice Malt	✓		✓	✓												✓				✓					
Rice Vinegar			✓									✓				✓						✓		✓	
Rosemary																✓		✓							
Rose Water																✓				✓	✓				
Rum																✓		✓						✓	
Saffron					✓							✓					✓			✓					
Scallion	✓	✓		✓								✓				✓			✓					✓	
Seafood													✓							✓					✓
Sea Salt		✓	✓			✓	✓						✓												✓
Seitan															✓					✓					
Sesame Oil			✓												✓					✓					
Sesame Seed						✓			✓								✓			✓					
Sherry																✓			✓	✓				✓	
Snow Peas			✓	✓													✓			✓					
Soy Milk																	✓			✓					
Soy Sauce			✓	✓		✓							✓												✓

MERIDIANS ROUTES   ENERGIES   FLAVOURS

FOODS, ENERGIES AND FLAVOURS

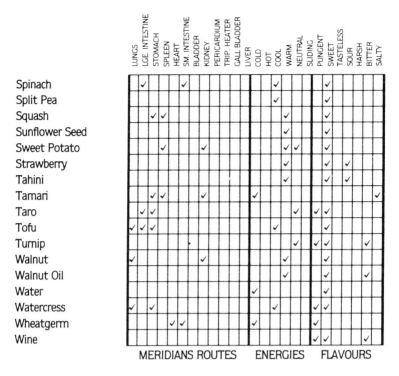

ACTIONS OF FOODS IN THE SEASONAL RECIPES

WINTER

Recipe	Energetic Actions
Baked Fish Rolls with Tofu Filling	Warming/hot/tonifies *Ki* and blood
Broccoli Cauliflower Mousseline	Tones *Ki* and Blood; Lubricates Dryness
Broccoli with Black Bean Sauce	Expels wind; tonifies *Ki* and blood
Buckwheat with Fennel, Onions and Mushrooms	Tonifies *Ki* and blood
Carrots in Orange Juice	Cool
Endive, Radish and Mandarin Salad	Cooling
Layered Vegetable Casserole	Warming
Parsnip Pie	Warming
Spiced Chickpeas (without Topping)	Expels cold; removes blood stagnation
Spinach Garlic Soup	Tonifies *Ki* and blood
Split Pea Soup	Dries damp
Snow pea Arame Salad	Cooling (softens hardness)
Vinaigrette Dressing (for Snow Pea Salad)	Warm

SPRING

Almond Potato Puffs	Tonifies *Ki* and Blood
Apricot Leek Crepes	Lubricates dryness; tonifies *Ki* and blood;
Basil Chicken	Tonifies *Ki* and blood; expels cold
Bean Salad	(Kidney) tonifies *Ki* and blood
Broad Bean Salad	Tonifies *Ki* and blood; eliminates water retention
Buddha's Casserole	Cooling, clears heat; tonifies *Ki* and blood
Eggplant Orientale	Tonifies *Ki* and blood; clears heat

Dilled Leek and Zucchini Soup	Removes stagnant blood; expels cold; regulates *Ki*
Mustard Pickles	Counteracts toxins
Spring Fish Tarts	Tonifies *Ki* and blood; lubricates dryness
Walnut Vegetable Salad	Tonifies *Ki* and blood; clears heat, expels cold

SUMMER

Recipe	**Energetic Actions**
Aduki Bean Rolls	Tonifies *Ki* and blood; removes damp
Bitter Green Salad	Tonifies *Ki* and blood
Coconut Fish Teriyaki	Expels cold, clears heat; tonifies *Ki*; produces fluids
Creamy Chicken Lasagne	Tonifies *Ki* and blood; clears heat; nourishes heart; removes blood stagnation
Five Heaps Noodles	Clears heat, expels cold; tonifies *Ki*
Gingered Noodle Soup	Relieves summer heat; tonifies *Ki* and blood
Lemon Zucchini and Olives	Produces fluids; expels cold; tonifies *Ki* and blood
Mixed Pepper Salad	Dries damp; detoxicant; tonifies *Ki*
Moroccan Vegetable Salad	Tonifies *Ki* and blood; clears heat; expels cold
Stuffed Golden Nuggets	Expels cold; produces fluid; tonifies *Ki* and blood
Summer Kebabs	Promotes energy circulation; tonifies *Ki* and blood
Tofu Loaf	Tonifies *Ki* and blood

LATE SUMMER

Recipe	**Energetic Actions**
Bulghur Timbales	Tonifies *Ki* and blood; clears heat
Butternut Spice	Dries damp; tonifies *Ki* and blood
Chickpea Macadamia Soup	Tonifies *Ki* and blood
Coconut Prawns	Tonifies *Ki* and blood; expels cold; promotes lactation (prawns)

Corn and Rice Combo	Tonifies *Ki* and blood
Fig and Endive Salad	Tonifies *Ki* and blood; dries damp
Fish Exotica	Tonifies *Ki* and blood
Millet and Split Pea Loaf	Tonifies *Ki* and blood
Sesame Spinach	Clears heat; tonifies *Ki* and blood; lubricates dryness
Spinach Crowns and Ginger Stir Fry	Tonifies *Ki* and blood
Vegetable Kebabs	Tonifies *Ki* and blood
Vegetable Tofu Quiche	Clears heat, tonifies *Ki* and blood

AUTUMN

Chestnut Rice	Tonifies *Ki* and blood; relieves diarrhoea
Chicken or Fish Balls	Tonifies *Ki* and blood; expels cold
Chicken or Fish Balls with Basil Sauce	Clears heat, expels cold; tonifies *Ki* and blood
Endive Beet Salad	Tonifies *Ki* and blood
Haricot Bean Hotpot	Tonifies *Ki* and blood
Leek Croquettes	Expels cold; benefits *Ki*
Lima Bean and Rosemary Soup	Tonifies *Ki* and blood
Olive Chestnut Patties	Tonifies *Ki* and blood
Oriental Salad	Tonifies *Ki* and blood; clears heat
Peanut Pumpkin Fritters	Tonifies *Ki* and blood; harmonizes the Stomach
Fresh Coriander Sauce (for Peanut Pumpkin Fritters)	Tonifies *Ki* and blood
Walnut Broccoli	Tonifies *Ki* and blood; expels cold
Watercress Miso Soup	Expel cold; removes Blood stagnation; clears heat

BREAKFASTS

Congee

Aduki Bean Congee	Removes damp; useful in edema and gout
Apricot Kernel Congee	Good for asthma and coughs
Carrot Congee	Good for indigestion and chronic dysentery
Celery Congee	Cooling

A C T I O N S   O F   F O O D S

Chestnut (dried) Congee	Strengthens lower back and knees; tonifies kidneys
Date and Ginger Congee	Sedates and calms the spirit; strengthens the digestion; promotes circulation of *Ki* and blood
Dry Ginger Congee	Cold and deficient digestive problems such as anorexia, vomiting and diarrhoea and indigestion
Fennel Congee	Cures *Ki* stagnation, carmative
Leek Congee	Warming and tonifying; good for chronic diarrhoea
Ming Bean Congee	Cools summer heat
Pine Nut Congee	Harmonizes large intestines; useful in wind dis-eases
Radish Congee	Cools hot problems of digestive organs
Spinach Congee	Sedative
Taro Root Congee	Tonifying and nutritive
Wheat Berry Congee	Cooling, calming and sedative

Adapted from *Prince Wen Hui's Cook, Chinese Dietary Therapy,* by Bob Flaws and Honora Wolfe, Paradigm Publications, Brookline Ma. 1983

Note: Many foods are listed as tonifying the *Ki* and Blood. This is an energetic way of describing the food to be nourishing and nutritive.

If a group of principles appear together, such as 'Removes stagnant blood, expels cold, regulates *Ki*', this means that the food activates both Blood and *Ki* circulation, relieves congestion and stagnation and improves function.

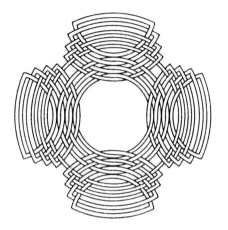

SUITABILITY OF THE RECIPES FOR VARIOUS DIETS

Denotes the use of tamari where tamari/shoyu is indicated in the recipe. (Tamari is wheat-free; shoyu contains wheat)

WINTER RECIPES

	NON-DAIRY	VEGAN	RAW	GLUTEN FREE	CANDIDA	PRITIKIN
Baked Fish Rolls with Tofu Filling	✓			✓		
Broccoli with Black Bean Sauce	✓	✓		✓		
Broccoli Cauliflower Mousseline				✓		
Broccoli Cauliflower Mousseline (Lemon Tamari Sauce)	✓	✓	✓	✓*		✓
Buckwheat with Fennel, Onions and Mushrooms				✓		
Carrots in Orange Juice	✓	✓		✓		
Endive, Radish and Mandarin Salad	✓	✓	✓	✓	✓	✓
Endive, Radish and Mandarin Salad (Tofu Dressing)	✓	✓	✓	✓		
Layered Vegetable Casserole	✓	✓		✓*		
Parsnip Pie (Filling)				✓		
Parsnip Pie (Pastry)	✓	✓				
Spiced Chickpeas	✓	✓		✓		
Spiced Chickpeas (Mochi Topping)	✓	✓				

MACROBIOTICS & BEYOND

	NON-DAIRY	VEGAN	RAW	GLUTEN FREE	CANDIDA	PRITIKIN
Spinach Garlic Soup	✓	✓		✓		
Split Pea Soup	✓	✓		✓*		✓
Snow Pea Arame Salad	✓	✓		✓	✓	
Snow Pea Arame Salad (Vinaigrette Dressing)			✓	✓		

SPRING RECIPES

	NON-DAIRY	VEGAN	RAW	GLUTEN FREE	CANDIDA	PRITIKIN
Almond Potato Puffs						
Apricot Leek Crepes (Crepes)						
Apricot Leek Crepes (Filling)	✓					
Apricot Leek Crepes (Green Sauce)	✓	✓	✓	✓	✓	
Basil Chicken	✓			✓		✓
Basil Chicken (Spring Mayonnaise)	✓	✓	✓	✓		
Basil Chicken (Sesame Ginger Toasts)	✓	✓				
Bean Salad	✓	✓		✓	✓	✓
Bean Salad (Miso Dressing)	✓	✓	✓	✓		
Broad Bean Salad	✓	✓		✓		
Broad Bean Salad (Vinegar Dressing)	✓	✓	✓	✓*		

RECIPES FOR VARIOUS DIETS

	NON-DAIRY	VEGAN	RAW	GLUTEN FREE	CANDIDA	PRITIKIN
Buddha's Casserole	✓	✓				✓
Buddha's Casserole (Braising Liquid)	✓	✓		✓*		
Eggplant Orientale (Sauce)				✓		
Dilled Leek and Zucchini Soup	✓	✓		✓	✓	
Mustard Pickles	✓	✓	✓	✓		
Spring Fish Tarts (Pastry)	✓			✓	✓	✓
Spring Fish Tarts (Tofu Nut Cream)	✓	✓	✓	✓		
Spring Fish Tarts (Vegetable Filling)	✓	✓		✓		
Walnut Vegetable Salad	✓	✓		✓		✓
Walnut Vegetable Salad (Dressing)	✓	✓	✓	✓		

MACROBIOTICS & BEYOND

SUMMER RECIPES

	NON-DAIRY	VEGAN	RAW	GLUTEN FREE	CANDIDA	PRITIKIN
Aduki Bean Rolls	✓	✓		✓		
Bitter Green Salad (Dressing)	✓	✓	✓	✓		
Coconut Fish Teriyaki	✓			✓		
Creamy Chicken Lasagne (Chicken Sauce)	✓			✓		
Creamy Chicken Lasagne (Mushrooms)	✓			✓		
Five Heaps Noodles	✓	✓		✓		✓
Five Heaps Noodles (Dressing)	✓	✓	✓	✓*		
Gingered Noodle Soup	✓	✓		*		
Lemon Zucchini and Olives	✓	✓	✓	✓	✓	
Mixed Pepper Salad (Dressing)	✓	✓	✓	✓		
Moroccan Vegetable Salad	✓	✓				
Stuffed Golden Nuggets				✓		
Summer Kebabs (Marinade)	✓	✓		✓*		
Tofu Loaf	✓	✓		✓*		
Tofu Loaf (Almond Milk)	✓	✓		✓		
Tofu Loaf (Sauce)	✓	✓				
Whole Vegetables on the Grill	✓	✓		✓	✓	✓

176

RECIPES FOR VARIOUS DIETS

LATE SUMMER RECIPES

	NON-DAIRY	VEGAN	RAW	GLUTEN FREE	CANDIDA	PRITIKIN
Bulghur Timbales	✓	✓				
Butternut Spice	✓	✓		✓		
Chickpea Macadamia Soup	✓	✓		✓		
Coconut Prawns (Batter)	✓	✓		✓		✓
Coconut Prawns (Peach Relish)	✓	✓	✓	✓		
Corn and Rice Combo	✓	✓		*		
Fig and Endive Salad	✓	✓	✓	✓		✓
Fig and Endive Salad (Dressing)	✓	✓	✓	✓		
Fish Exotica	✓			✓		
Fish Exotica (Sauce)	✓			*		
Millet and Split Pea Loaf	✓	✓		✓		
Sesame Spinach	✓	✓		✓*		
Spinach Crowns and Ginger Stir Fry	✓	✓				
Vegetable Kebabs (Marinade)	✓	✓		✓		
Vegetable Tofu Quiche (Filling)	✓	✓		✓		
Vegetable Tofu Quick (Pastry)	✓	✓				✓

MACROBIOTICS & BEYOND

AUTUMN RECIPES

	NON-DAIRY	VEGAN	RAW	GLUTEN FREE	CANDIDA	PRITIKIN
Chestnut Rice	✓	✓		✓	✓	✓
Chicken or Fish Balls				✓		
Chicken or Fish Balls (Basil Sauce)	✓	✓		✓		
Endive Beet Salad	✓	✓		✓	✓	✓
Endive Beet Salad (Orange Caraway Vinaigrette)	✓	✓	✓	✓		
Haricot Bean Hot pot	✓	✓		✓		
Leek Croquettes						✓
Leek Croquettes (Chili Dip)	✓	✓	✓	✓*		✓
Lime Bean and Rosemary Soup	✓	✓		✓	✓	✓
Olive Chestnut Patties	✓	✓		✓		
Oriental Salad	✓	✓		✓*		
Oriental Salad (Dressing)	✓	✓	✓	✓		
Peanut Pumpkin Fritters	✓	✓		✓		
Peanut Pumpkin Fritters (Fresh Coriander Sauce)	✓	✓		✓*		✓
Walnut Broccoli (Sauce)	✓	✓		✓*		
Watercress Miso Soup	✓	✓		✓		✓

RECIPES FOR VARIOUS DIETS

COLD DESSERTS

	NON-DAIRY	VEGAN	RAW	GLUTEN FREE	CANDIDA	PRITIKIN
Cherry Carob Pudding	✓	✓		✓		
Fruit Freezes	✓	✓	✓	✓		✓
Soy Custard				✓		
Strawberry Mousse				✓		

FRESH FRUIT DESSERTS

	NON-DAIRY	VEGAN	RAW	GLUTEN FREE	CANDIDA	PRITIKIN
Annie's Peaches	✓	✓		✓		
Apple Pear Walnut Crisp (Fruit Mixture)	✓	✓		✓		
Apple Pear Walnut Crisp (Topping)	✓	✓				
Stuffed Ginger Apples	✓	✓		✓		
Summer Berries	✓	✓	✓	✓		

MACROBIOTICS & BEYOND

TARTS, PUFFS AND OTHER SWEET DELIGHTS

	NON-DAIRY	VEGAN	RAW	GLUTEN FREE	CANDIDA	PRITIKIN
Blueberry Cream Pie (Pastry	✓					
Blueberry Cream Pie (Filling)				✓		
Blueberry Cream Pie (Topping)	✓	✓		✓		
Fruit Tart (Pastry)						
Fruit Tart (Filling)				✓		
Fruit Tart Glaze	✓	✓		✓		

OTHERS

	NON-DAIRY	VEGAN	RAW	GLUTEN FREE	CANDIDA	PRITIKIN
Carob Fudge	✓	✓		✓		
Oatmeal Cinnamon Puffs						
Sweet Puffs	✓					
Sweet Puffs (Glaze)	✓	✓		✓		
Walnut or Almond Balls	✓	✓	✓	✓		
Walnut Bean Puffs (Filling)	✓	✓		✓		
Walnut Bean Puffs (Pastry)	✓	✓		✓		

RECIPES FOR VARIOUS DIETS

CAKES

	NON-DAIRY	VEGAN	RAW	GLUTEN FREE	CANDIDA	PRITIKIN
Apple Walnut Cake						
Bo's Sixth Birthday Cake						
Bo's Sixth Birthday Cake (Carob Icing)	✓		✓	✓		
Carrot and Sultana Cake						
Julie's Cake				✓		
Julie's Cake (Topping)				✓		
Pear and Pine Nut Supreme Cake	✓	✓				
Pear and Pine Nut Supreme Cake (Pear Topping)	✓	✓		✓		
Pear and Pine Nut Supreme Cake (Coating)	✓	✓		✓		✓

181

MACROBIOTICS & BEYOND

COOKIES, BISCUITS and BARS

	NON-DAIRY	VEGAN	RAW	GLUTEN FREE	CANDIDA	PRITIKIN
Apple Macaroon Slices (Crust)	✓	✓				
Apple Macaroon Slices (Topping)						
Big Spoon Cookies				✓		
Date Nut Bars (Crust)	✓	✓				
Date Nut Bars (Filling)	✓	✓		✓		✓
Everyone's Favourite Biscuit	✓	✓				
Five Spice Cookies						
Fruit and Nut Squares	✓	✓				
Ginger Drops						
Great Big Ones	✓	✓				
Nut Rounds	✓	✓				
Yellow Diamonds						

182

RECIPES FOR VARIOUS DIETS

BREAKFAST RECIPES

	NON-DAIRY	VEGAN	RAW	GLUTEN FREE	CANDIDA	PRITIKIN
Casserole Special				*		
Congee	✓	✓		✓	✓	✓
Foccacia for Friends	✓	✓				
Four Seasons Jam	✓	✓		✓		✓
Oat Almond Pikelets	✓	✓				
Olive Peasant Bread						
Potato Pancakes with Poached Eggs						
Rolled Pancakes						
Soy Spritzers	✓	✓	✓	✓		✓
Spinach Crepes (Crepes)						
Spinach Crepes (Filling)	✓	✓		✓		
Spinach Crepes (Sauce)	✓	✓		✓		
Strawberry Pancakes						
Strawberry Pancakes (Filling)	✓	✓		✓		
Sunday Loaf	✓	✓				
Sweet Corn Popovers						
Tasty Spreads: Hazelnut Miso Spread	✓	✓		✓		

	NON-DAIRY	VEGAN	RAW	GLUTEN FREE	CANDIDA	PRITIKIN
Onion Butter	✓	✓		✓		
Rainbow Spread	✓	✓	✓	✓		
Sunshine Spread	✓	✓		✓		✓

BEVERAGES

	NON-DAIRY	VEGAN	RAW	GLUTEN FREE	CANDIDA	PRITIKIN
Apple, Pear and Lemon Smoothie	✓	✓	✓	✓		✓
Berry Soymilk Shake	✓	✓	✓	✓		
Daniel's Winter Warmer	✓	✓		✓		
Hot Orange Tea	✓	✓		✓		
Spiced Tea	✓	✓		✓		

RECIPES FOR VARIOUS DIETS

STOCKS

	NON-DAIRY	VEGAN	RAW	GLUTEN FREE	CANDIDA	PRITIKIN
'Anything Goes' Stock	✓			✓	✓	✓
Basic White Fish Stock	✓			✓		✓
Chicken Stock	✓			✓		✓
Dashi Stock	✓	✓		✓	✓	✓
Noddle Water Stock	✓	✓				✓
Porridge Stock	✓	✓				✓
Whole Grain Stock	✓	✓				✓

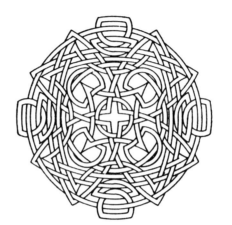

ALTERNATIVE INGREDIENTS FOR VARIOUS DIETARY REQUIREMENTS

When you are selecting recipes please note that there are choices given for some of the ingredients. This allows those people who have certain food intolerances or dietary restrictions to choose an appropriate food. Where choices are not given in the ingredients listed in the recipe, you may find it useful to consult the following list.

ARROWROOT (1 tablespoon) = 2 teaspoons kuzu powder

BAKING POWDER (1 teaspoon) = $1/3$ teaspoon baking soda plus $2/3$ teaspoon cream of tartar and ¼ teaspoon arrowroot

BROWN RICE VINEGAR (1 tablespoon) = 2 teaspoons lemon juice

CHESTNUT FLOUR = any *one* of the following:
4 parts brown rice flour and 1 part soy flour, or 4 parts oat flour and 1 part soy flour, or 4 parts barley flour and 1 part oat flour

CHOCOLATE (30 g) = 3 tablespoons carob powder plus 1 tablespoon oil

COCOA = carob powder in equal measure

CORNSTARCH (1 tablespoon) = 4 teaspoons wholewheat flour, or 1 teaspoon arrowroot or   kuzu; in sauces use $1/3$ cup arrowroot for 1 cup cornstarch

CREAM = yoghurt in equal measure

EGGS N.B. (Egg white acts as leavening, egg yolk as a binder)
As a binder: 1 egg = 1 teaspoon nut butter (tahini, cashew, almond, etc.) with water or fruit juice to consistency of whipped egg, or 1 part soy flour and 2 parts water blended and heated (thickens as it cools)

As a leavening agent: 1 egg = 1 teaspoon baking powder or ½ teaspoon arrowroot plus ¼ teaspoon baking soda or 2 egg whites stiffly beaten

As a binder and leavener: 2 eggs = 4 tablespoons almond or cashew butter with 2 tablespoons lemon juice or 1 tablespoon vinegar

For cookies or biscuits: 4 eggs = 1 tablespoon oil, 2 tablespoons baking powder substitute and 2 tablespoons water or fruit juice

MIRIN/RICE WINE (1 tablespoon) = 1 tablespoon sweet sherry

MILK = Soymilk, nut milk or coconut milk in equal measure

MISO (1 tablespoon) = ½ teaspoon sea salt

PEANUT BUTTER = almond, cashew, sunflower, hazelnut, sesame or tahini butter in equal measure

SEA SALT (1 teaspoon) = ½ teaspoon dried kelp powder

MACROBIOTICS & BEYOND

SHOYU or TAMARI (2 teaspoons) = ¼ teaspoon sea salt, or 1 tablespoon miso (salty) or

2 tablespoons white or natto miso (sweeter)

UMEBOSHI PLUMS (1 tablespoon) = 1 tablespoon chopped capers and ½ teaspoon sea salt

WHOLEWHEAT FLOUR (1 cup) = ½ cup arrowroot and ½ cup soy flour, or any *one* of the following: ¾ cup brown rice flour, 1 cup corn flour, 1¼ cups barley flour, ¾ cup potato flour, 1⅓ cups oat flour (or rolled oats finely ground), 1⅓ cups soy flour

ALTERNATIVE SWEETENERS

When I prepare desserts, I usually choose a sweetener according to what kind of taste, texture and degree of sweetness I would like.

This list is designed to help you substitute one natural sweetener for another, and experiment in terms of the different effects they produce. Remember, always decrease or increase the amount of liquid or flour in the recipe according to the liquid content of the sweetener.

In all recipes, ½ cup sweetener = ½ cup maple syrup
½ cup honey
⅓ cup molasses
½ cup black sugar
½ cup coconut sugar
1¼ cups maltose*
1½ cups barley malt extract*
½ cup fruit juice concentrate
sugarless fruit jam or jelly*
1¼ cups dried fruit purée**
1¼ cups brown rice malt syrup*
2 cups fruit juice or ½ fruit and ½ carrot juice*
½ cup unsweetened frozen juice concentrate
(e.g., orange juice)*

— These sweeteners are all gluten free, except for the maltose and barley malt extract which cannot be used if following a gluten-free diet.

— When using any sweetener in place of sugar in an ordinary recipe, reduce liquid content in recipe by ¼ cup or more, depending on the sweetener you choose. If no liquid is called for in the recipe, add 3 – 5 tablespoons of flour for each ¾ cup of sweetener.

— Be sure to heat maltose, malt or brown rice malt syrup before working with it.

— Oil the measuring cup and spoon before measuring liquid sweeteners.

— When maltose, brown rice malt syrup or barley malt extract is used, it may liquefy the consistency of the mixture. This is more likely to occur when eggs are not used. To compensate, use more dry ingredients.

— Those liquid sweeteners which have an acid factor (honey, molasses) need neutralising by the addition of baking soda.

— Look for fruits that have been sun-dried rather than oven-dried if using dried fruit for a sweetener or in any recipe. Most dried fruits these days have been treated with sulphur dioxide gas or powdered sulphur bisulfite during the drying process. Commercial raisins and sultanas are usually dipped in potassium carbonate solution before drying. Once dried, potassium sorbate is added as a preservative. Most dried fruits are sprayed with mineral oil or liquid paraffin to prevent them from sticking to each other. All of these are really unnecessary.

* If these sweeteners are used, the amount of liquid will have to be reduced or the amount of dry ingredients will have to be increased. Add ground nuts, seeds, coconut or carob flour or arrowroot for best results.
** Includes the following: nectarines, peaches, apricots, prunes, pears, apples, mangoes, paw-paws, raisins, sultanas, currants, figs, dates, Chinese dates, pineapples, and bananas.

EQUIVALENCY CHART

AGAR-AGAR (1 bar) = 4 – 6 tablespoons agar-agar flakes, or ½ tablespoon powder (later not recommended for use)

BASIL, freshly chopped (2 tablespoons) = 1 teaspoon dried basil and 1½ tablespoons freshly chopped parsley leaves

CINNAMON (2½ teaspoons) = 1 cinnamon stick

GARLIC, concentrated (1 teaspoon) = 2 cloves fresh garlic

HERBS, dried (¼ teaspoon) = 2 tablespoons fresh herbs

LEMON JUICE (1½ tablespoons) = ½ medium-sized lemon

NUT MILK (1 cup) = 1 cup hot water or fruit juice and 2 tablespoons any nut butter such as almond, cashew, hazelnut or sunflower seed

SPINACH OR OTHER LEAFY GREENS, chopped (4 cups) = ½ bunch

WHOLEWHEAT FLOUR (1 cup minus 2 tablespoons) = 1 cup white flour

YEAST, dry (2 teaspoons) = 30 g fresh yeast

METRIC CONVERSION CHARTS

TABLESPOONS AND OUNCES	GRAMS
1 pinch = less than ⅛ teaspoon (dry)	0.5 gram
1 dash = 3 drops to ¼ teaspoon (liquid)	1.25 grams
1 teaspoon (liquid)	5.0 grams
3 teaspoons = 1 tablespoon = ½ ounce	14.3 grams
2 tablespoons = 1 ounce	28.35 grams
4 tablespoons = 2 ounces = ¼ cup	56.7 grams
8 tablepsoons = 4 ounces = ½ cup (1 stick of butter) . . .	113.4 grams
8 tablespoons (flour) = about 2 ounces	72.0 grams
16 tablespoons = 8 ounces = 1 cup = ½ pound	226.8 grams
32 tablespoons = 16 ounces = 2 cups = 1 pound	453.6 grams or 0.4536 kilogram
64 tablespoons = 32 ounces = 1 quart = 2 pounds	907.0 grams or 0.907 kilogram
1 quart = roughly 1 litre	

TEMPERATURES: °FAHRENHEIT (F) TO °CELSIUS (C)

-10°F = -23.3°C (freezer storage)	300°F = 148.8°C
0°F = -17.7°C	325°F = 162.8°C
32°F = 0°C (water freezes)	350°F = 177°C (baking)
50°F = 10°C	375°F = 190.5°C
68°F = 20°C (room temperature)	400°F = 204.4°C (hot oven)
100°F = 37.7°C	425°F = 218.3°C
150°F = 65.5°C	450°F = 232°C (very hot oven)
205°F = 96.1°C (water simmers)	475°F = 246.1°C
212°F = 100°C (water boils)	500°F = 260°C (broiling)

CONVERSION FACTORS

ounces to grams: multiply ounce figure by 28.3 to get number of grams
grams to ounces: multiply gram figure by .0353 to get number of ounces
pounds to grams: multiply pound figure by 453.59 to get number of grams
pounds to kilograms: multiply pound figure by 0.45 to get number of kilograms
ounces to millilitres: multiply ounce figure by 30 to get number of millilitres
cups to litres: multiply cup figure by 0.24 to get number of litres
Fahrenheit to Celsius: subtract 32 from the Fahrenheit figure, multiply by 5, then divide by 9 to get Celsius figure

METRIC CONVERSION CHARTS

Celsius to Fahrenheit: multiply Celsius figure by 9, divide by 5, then add 32 to get Fahrenheit figure

inches to centimetres: multiply inch figure by 2.54 to get number of centimetres

centimetres to inches: multiply centimetre figure by .39 to get number of inches

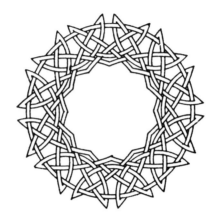

GLOSSARY

AGAR-AGAR

Otherwise known as *kanten*, agar-agar is a setting agent composed of a variety of different sea vegetables. They are soaked and washed, simmered and pressed. The liquid that comes off is put into shallow boxes and hardens. It is then dried again and the process is repeated for several days. It can be used exactly like gelatin, but needs to be cooked or simmered for several minutes before setting. It provides iron, phosphorus, calcium, and vitamins A, B1, B6, B12, biotin, C, D and K.

ARAME

A thin, black, thread-like sea vegetable often used as a side dish or tossed in salads or rice. It is similar in texture and appearance to *hijiki* sea vegetable, and is rich in iron, calcium and other minerals.

ARROWROOT

Similar to *kuzu* and cornstarch, this thickening agent can be used in soups, gravies, cookies, cakes and custards.

BROWN RICE VINEGAR

A mild-tasting vinegar made from brown rice. Pure brown rice vinegar is very high in amino acids and has all of the ten essential amino acids. Because of the high content of amino acids in brown rice vinegar, it can dissolve a build-up of lactic acid in the body. (The over-consumption of acid-forming foods such as animal fats, sugars and refined grains, as well as excessive periods of mental or physical exertion, leads to a heightened presence of lactic acid in the blood and tissues of the body. This can create a feeling of nervousness and ill-tempered irritation, or if lactic acid combines with protein to create lactic acid protein in the body cells, muscle stiffening and fatigue may result). Fruit vinegars contain a smaller amount of amino acids, and ordinary vinegars and synthetic vinegars have no amino acids at all.

CAROB FLOUR

Otherwise known as St John's bread, this food is an ideal natural substitute in recipes calling for the use of cocoa or chocolate. The flavour and colour it imparts is similar to that of chocolate, yet it does not contain calcium oxylate, theobromine and caffeine which are in products made from the cocoa bean.

MACROBIOTICS & BEYOND

CHICKPEA FLOUR (BESAN)
Used a great deal in Indian cuisine, this flour makes a good addition to any pantry. It can be used in breads, biscuits, sauces and batters, and is gluten free.

CHINESE BLACK MUSHROOMS (SHIITAKE)
These exotic mushrooms are found in Asian shops stocking Chinese and Japanese foodstuffs. They are used in soups, stocks, vegetable dishes, salads, and are effective in helping the body neutralise the effects of excessive consumption of animal fats and salt.
(CLOUD EARS: see MUSHROOMS, MO-ER)

COUSCOUS
Couscous, the national dish of Morocco, Algeria and Tunisia, is traditionally served in steaming mounds with stews. It is made from semolina, which has been steamed and rolled, and can be used in savoury as well as sweet dishes.

DAMP (EXTERNAL)
Damp usually arises from the environment, such as very wet weather for a long period of time. Some of the signs of damp are the body feels heavy, the head feels dull and vague, and the memory is affected.

DAMP (INTERNAL)
This is usually caused by a weakening of the digestive system due to overeating or eating inappropriate foods for your own internal condition. Also it can arise from the use of too many drugs or stimulants such as coffee. Some accompaning symptoms are worry, abdominal swelling, lethargy and fatigue.

NOTE: Both damp and dry conditions are part of the six energetic phases and not the eight divisions which include *Yin* and *Yang*, Internal and External, Hot and Cold, Deficiency and Excess. However, they have been included for practical reasons, as it is a good diagnostic tool when you want to determine your condition.

DEFICIENCY
Usually a deficiency is chronic in nature, and is characterised by insufficient Blood, *Ki*, or other substances. It can also manifest, if there is underactivity in any of the *Yang* or *Yin* aspects of the organs. Some of the symptoms that can be produced are weak and frail movement; pale, sallow or ashen face colour; spontaneous sweating; pain that is relieved by pressure; dizziness, etc.

DRY
See Chinese System of Diagnosis and Treatment.

GLOSSARY

EXCESS
This particular pattern is generally exhibited when some bodily function becomes overactive, or when there is an obstruction thus causing an accumulation of *Ki* or Blood for example. It can also come about when some external condition such as too much damp or cold weather comes about. Some symptoms of Excess are; loud and full voice; heavy breathing; scanty urination; abdominal pains that get worse when pressure is used on them; Generally speaking, Excess patterns tend to be acute in nature.

FERMENTED BLACK BEANS
This is a wonderful seasoning agent consisting of black beans which have been preserved in a salty brine, then dried, fermented and packaged (sometimes with dried ginger root). They should be rinsed before being used, and although quite salty on their own they tend to lend a delicate flavour when used in seafood, poultry or vegetable dishes. They can be kept indefinitely in a tightly covered jar, needing no refrigeration.

JAPANESE PEPPER (SEVEN-SPICE PEPPER)
This spicy pepper is a delicious blend of ground orange peel, hot red pepper, *sansho* pepper, hemp seeds, sesame seeds, ground *nori* seaweed and poppy seeds. It is used as a seasoning and condiment, and is available in Japanese food shops.

Ki
Ki is the source of all movement in the body and accompanies all movement, and is inseparable from movement. In the body, *Ki* is in constant motion and has four primary directions: entering, leaving, descending and ascending. *Ki* is also the source of harmonious transformation in the body. For example when food is taken into the body, it is then transformed into other substances such as sweat, urine, blood, tears and *Ki* itself. *Ki* also maintains the normal heat in the body or in any part of the body.

DEFICIENT Ki
This is when there is insufficient *Ki* to perform any one of the five *Ki* functions. It can affect the whole body producing symptoms such as lethargy and a lack of desire to move, or it can affect an organ such as the kidneys, which will produce symptoms such as edema.

STAGNANT Ki
This means that the *Ki* cannot move smoothly through the body, and it can manifest itself in the organs, limbs (pain) and meridians (aches in the body). If the lungs become affected symptoms can arise such as a cough.

MACROBIOTICS & BEYOND

KOMBU
A large, broad, flat, dark green sea vegetable, *kombu* grows in the deepest part of the ocean. Rich in essential minerals, it is mainly used in soup stocks and condiments, and can be cooked with beans and other vegetables.

KUZU
A white starch made from the root of a Japanese plant, *kuzu* (sometimes referred to as *kudzu*) is similar in properties to arrowroot and cornstarch. It is used for thickening soups, sauces, gravies and desserts, and is also used medicinally.

LEMON PEPPER, JAPANESE
Japan produces some of the best condiments in the world, particularly lemon pepper, which is made from a special pepper plant with a hint of a lemon flavour. It can be used in place of pepper, although it is nowhere near as spicy.

LOTUS SEEDS
These are small, pale yellowish seeds which come from the lotus plant and are available dried, with the skin on or blanched. Used for desserts in Chinese cuisine, they can also be used in vegetable dishes and soups.

MAPLE SYRUP
Maple syrup is tapped from the maple tree in North America and Canada. It takes 200 litres of maple sap to produce 4 litres of syrup. It is a completely natural food containing phosphorus, potassium and sodium, and has considerably more minerals than other types of refined sweeteners.

MIDDLE BURNER
This term refers to the stomach/spleen area in the body.

MIRIN
Mirin is a relative of sake. In the case of mirin, sweet rice is mixed with the wine, and after lengthy fermentation it is pressed and aged again for six months to two years in ceramic containers. Many brands of mirin, especially those sold in Asian food stores, are not naturally brewed and are sweetened with added sugar or corn syrup. Most of the mirin available in natural food stores is of a high quality, naturally fermented and authentic. Check the label to be sure.

MISO
A fermented bean paste made with soybeans, barley, rice, rice honey and kombu, *miso* is high in protein and vitamin B12, and is especially beneficial to the digestive and circulatory systems.

GLOSSARY

MOCHI
Mochi is made from sweet brown rice, pounded to a sticky dough then formed into small blocks and dried. When cooked these cakes soften and puff up, becoming delectably moist and chewy. *Mochi* makes great snacks, savoury or sweet. Stuff with sauces, or top with jam or maple syrup like waffles.

MUSHROOMS, MO-ER (CLOUD EARS)
A specialty of Szechuan province in China, this crinkly tree fungus is usually soaked in hot water for at least 30 minutes. The mushrooms should be rinsed well to remove sand, and the hard centre removed. They are best known for their texture and combine well with any ingredient.

NORI
Otherwise known as purple laver, *nori* consists of thin, paperlike sheets of dried seaweed used in soups and rice dishes, and for wrapping foods. It is available at most Asian food stores and can be kept indefinitely if kept well wrapped and refrigerated.

NUT MILK
For those of us who have an allergic reaction or an aversion to cow's or goat's milk, nut milk is a good alternative. It is made by lightly toasting skinned nuts, and blending them with warm juice or water and other seasonings till creamy and smooth. Sometimes it can be strained if desired.

RICE WINE, CHINESE
Rice wine is a yellowish grain wine, used like white, red or Japanese sweet wine (mirin) in cooking. If Chinese rice wine is unavailable, substitute a Japanese sake, Scotch, or a dry, white vermouth.

ROSE WATER
Distilled from fragrant rose petals, rose water is used for both savoury and sweet dishes.

SEA SALT
This type of salt has been extracted from sea water and has been minimally refined. It contains small amounts of trace elements and has no additives.

SEITAN GLUTEN MEAT
This is also known as 'wheat' gluten, and can be cooked in a variety of ways, which resembles meat in texture. It can be made at home (for the adventurous) or can be purchased ready to eat in many health food stores.

SESAME OIL, ROASTED
Thick and light brown in colour, sesame oil has a wonderful aroma and is made by roasting sesame seeds and pressing them to extract the oil — the thicker it is the better the flavour. Sesame oil is used as a seasoning more than in cooking because it burns too easily.

SEVEN SPICE PEPPER: see JAPANESE PEPPER

SHIITAKE: see CHINESE BLACK MUSHROOMS

SHOYU
This name is usually given to traditional, naturally fermented soy sauce to distinguish it from chemically processed varieties. *Shoyu* contains about 2 per cent more salt than *tamari*, and tastes slightly sweeter.

SOYMILK
Soy beverages, have become more and more popular over the past few years in Western societies. They are made from soybeans, which have been cooked and then mixed with various flavouring agents and contain small amounts of protein and calcium. Soymilk can be used in sauces, soups, gravies, custards, pies, cakes and puddings.

SOY SAUCE: see SHOYU and TAMARI

TAHINI
A smooth paste resembling peanut butter and made from ground, white sesame seeds. Can be used as a spread on bread when mixed with miso 4 to 1 or shoyu or tamari, or in salad dressings, soups, pates, pies, cakes, cookies or as a sauce over vegetables, or fish.

TAMARI
Like *shoyu, tamari* is a traditional, naturally fermented soy sauce (not chemically processed), but it is slightly less sweet than *shoyu*. Real tamari is made without the use of any wheat.

TOFU
Tofu made from soybeans is high in protein, low in fat, cholesterol and kilojoules. An ideal food for those of us who are watching our weight, it can be used in soups, vegetable dishes, dressings and desserts and is referred to as 'cheese' in the East.

G L O S S A R Y

TONIFY
To nourish, store and give sufficient nutritive energy.

UMEBOSHI
This type of pickled plum stimulates the appetite and digestion, and aids in maintaining an alkaline blood quality. They can be used for salad dressings and cooking vegetables for a salty sour flavour, or eaten (in suitable quantities) if you suffer from indigestion.

VINEGAR, BROWN RICE: see BROWN RICE VINEGAR

WAKAME
A long, thin sea vegetable, *wakame* can be used in soups, salads and vegetable dishes. High in iron, magnesium and iodine, it can be used in place of *kombu* for stock, or when baked dry it can be sprinkled on top of food for a condiment.

WIND
Wind, in nature is wandering, changeable, indefinite and indeterminable. When there is no particular dis-ease state but feelings of discomfort are apparent on the part of the patient, the diagnosis of wind is often used. Such common illnesses as the common cold, flu and even rheumatism or a type of arthritis can be referred to as evil wind. Eczema, is also a kind of damp wind that has succeeded to get out of the body by erupting through the skin.

YIN/YANG THEORY
'The logic underlying Chinese medical theory — a logic which assumes that a part can be understood only in its relation to the whole — can also be called synthetic or dialectical. In Chinese early naturalist and Taoist thought, this dialectical logic that explains relationships, patterns, and change is called Yin-Yang theory.' [1]

---

1. Kaptchuk, T.J. *The Web That has no Weaver*, Congdon and Weed, New York, 1983 page 7.

WHERE TO SHOP

Health Food Store Wholemeal flours, seeds, expeller-pressed unrefined oils, *miso*, *shoyu*, sea salt, *kuzu*, arrowroot, nut butters, unsulphured dried fruits, sweeteners, teas, grain coffee, fruit juices, bean curd *(tofu)*, soy milk, organic fruits and vegetables, free-range eggs, herbs, spices, natural flavourings, vitamin and mineral supplements, biodynamic goods, etc.

Asian Food Store (Japanese, Korean, Chinese) *Kuzu* flour, spices, herbs, maltose, nuts, seeds, oils, dried chestnuts, etc.

Middle Eastern Store Herbs, spices, grains, dried beans, tahini, nuts, seeds, olive oil, goat or sheep cheese, etc.

Italian Delicatessen Nuts, seeds, olive oil, grain, chestnut flour, fresh or dried herbs, etc.

Supermarkets Wholemeal flour, nuts, seeds, nut butters, herbs, spices, fruit juice, cider, honey, maple syrup, etc.

Not every item that you may wish to purchase may be found under one roof, but more and more items are being made available in local supermarkets and small shops. It will take time to familiarise yourself with where to find what, but this basic guide was designed with the expectation that natural food items will become more accessible in a number of places. If you can't find something, please ask for it. By creating a demand, the supply will automatically come! Experiment, and try something new. If you don't know how to use it, just ask your shopkeeper who will usually be more than willing to give advice.

BIBLIOGRAPHY

Butt, Gary, and Bloomfield, Frena, *Harmony Rules*, 1986, Arrow Books

Colbin, Annemarie, *Food and Healing*, 1986, Ballantine Books, New York

Davies, Dr. Stephen and Stewart, Dr Alan, *Nutritional Medicine*, 1987, Pan Books, London & Sydney

East Asian Medical Studies Society, The, *Fundamentals of Chinese Medicine*, 1985, Paradigm Publications, Brookline, Massachusetts

Ferré, Julia, *Basic Macrobiotic Cooking*, 1987, George Ohsawa Macrobiotic Foundation, Oroville, California

Flaws, Bob, and Wolfe, Honora, *Prince Wen Hui's Cook — Chinese Dietary Therapy*, 1983, Paradigm Publications, Brookline, Massachusetts

Haas, Elson M., M.D., *Staying Healthy With The Seasons*, 1981, Celestial Arts, Berkeley, California

Kaptchuk, T.J. O.M.D., *The Web That has no Weaver, Understanding Chinese Medicine*, Congdon and Weed, 1983, New York

Kavarana, Jenny, *Understanding Cookery*, 1979, MacMillan Press, Ltd

Kuo, Irene, *The Key to Chinese Cooking*, 1977, Nelson

Kushi, Aveline and Esko, Wendy, *Macrobiotic Family Favorites*, 1987, Japan Publications, Inc.

Kushi, Michio, *The Macrobiotic Way*, 1985, Avery Publishing Group Inc., Wayne, New Jersey

Lin, Hsiang Ju and Lin, Tsuifeng, *Chinese Gastronomy*, 1967, Harvest/HBJ

Lu, Henry C., *Chinese System of Food Cures*, 1986, Sterling Publishing Co. Inc., New York

Pearson, Mark, *The Companion Cookbook*, 1987, Doubleday, Sydney

Templeton, Louise, *The Right Food For Your Kids*, 1984, Century Publishing, London

Unschuld, P.U., *Medicine In China, A History Of Pharmaceutics*, 1986, University of California Press

Various, *Masterclass — Expert Lessons in Kitchen Skills*, 1982, Collins, Sydney